Power Yoga: Strength, Sweat, and Spirit

Leah Cullis

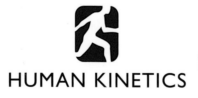

HUMAN KINETICS

Library of Congress Cataloging-in-Publication Data

Names: Cullis, Leah, 1980- author.
Title: Power yoga : strength, sweat, and spirit / Leah Cullis.
Description: Champaign, IL : Human Kinetics, [2019]
Identifiers: LCCN 2018017541 (print) | LCCN 2018018870 (ebook) | ISBN
   9781492560661 (ebook) | ISBN 9781492560654 (print)
Subjects: LCSH: Hatha yoga. | Mind and body.
Classification: LCC RA781.7 (ebook) | LCC RA781.7 .C844 2019 (print) | DDC
   613.7/046--dc23
LC record available at https://lccn.loc.gov/2018017541

ISBN: 978-1-4925-6065-4 (print)

Senior Acquisitions Editor: Michelle Maloney
Developmental Editor: Laura Pulliam
Managing Editor: Ann Gindes
Copyeditor: Michelle Horn
Senior Graphic Designer: Nancy Rasmus
Cover Designers: Keri Evans and Signe Higgins
Cover Design Associate: Susan Rothermel Allen
Photograph (cover): © Human Kinetics
Photographs (interior): © Human Kinetics unless otherwise noted
Photo Production Coordinator: Amy M. Rose
Photo Production Manager: Jason Allen
Printer: Versa Press

We thank Julianna Monceaux in Austin, Texas, for providing the location for the photo shoot for this book.

Human Kinetics books are available at special discounts for bulk purchase. Special editions or book excerpts can also be created to specification. For details, contact the Special Sales Manager at Human Kinetics.

Printed in the United States of America   10 9 8 7 6 5 4 3 2 1

The paper in this book is certified under a sustainable forestry program.

Human Kinetics
P.O. Box 5076
Champaign, IL 61825-5076
Website: www.HumanKinetics.com

In the United States, email info@hkusa.com or call 800-747-4457.
In Canada, email info@hkcanada.com.
In the United Kingdom/Europe, email hk@hkeurope.com.

For information about Human Kinetics' coverage in other areas of the world,
please visit our website: **www.HumanKinetics.com**

E7218

For my daughter Victoria, my
spirited and powerful teacher.

CONTENTS

Pose Finder   vi
Foreword   viii
Preface   x
Acknowledgments   xiv
Introduction   xvi

CHAPTER 1   **The Power of Yoga**   1
Yoga for Life Today   2
The Physical Practice   7

CHAPTER 2   **Intention**   15
Setting Your Intention   16
Cultivating Focus   22
Applying the Right Effort   26

CHAPTER 3   **Power Principles**   31
Breath   32
Foundation   37
Energy Locks   47
Chakras   49
Heat   52
Flow   56

CHAPTER 4   **Warm-Up Poses and Sequences**   61
Opening Poses   62
Warm-Up Poses   76
Opening Sequences   93
Vinyasa   98
Sun Salutations   100

CHAPTER 5   **Power Poses and Sequences**   115
Power Poses   116
Power Sequences   161

CHAPTER 6   **Peak Poses and Sequences**   169
Igniting Your Peak   170
Peak Poses   174
Peak Sequences   210

CHAPTER 7   **Cool-Down Poses and Sequences**   217

Power in Opposites   218

Hips   222

Forward Folds   234

Final Rest   238

Cool-Down Sequences   242

CHAPTER 8   **Core Strength Poses and Sequences**   245

Cultivating Core Strength   246

Core Poses   247

Core Sequences   254

CHAPTER 9   **Upper-Body Strength Sequences**   267

What Is Your Upper Body Saying?   268

Upper-Body Sequences   270

CHAPTER 10   **Lower-Body Strength Sequences**   283

Trust Your Foundation   284

Lower-Body Sequences   285

CHAPTER 11   **Yoga Within Your Other Workouts**   295

Power Yoga and Injury Prevention   296

Sport-Specific Yoga Sequences   297

CHAPTER 12   **Your Power Yoga Plan**   313

Get the Most Out of Your Practice   314

Your Power Yoga Plan: Sequences   317

About the Author   345

Earn Continuing Education Credits/Units   346

POSE FINDER

Chapter 4

Child's Pose	63	Downward-Facing Dog	80
Tabletop	64	Down Dog Splits	81
Cat and Cow	66	Halfway Lift	82
Reclined Bound Angle	68	Standing Forward Fold	83
Supine Twist	69	High Plank	85
Easy Pose	70	Low Plank	87
Thread the Needle	72	Upward-Facing Dog	88
Knees-to-Chest	73	Low Cobra	89
Rock 'n' Rolls	74	Chair Pose	90
Supported Hero Pose	75	Warrior I	91
Mountain Pose	77		

Chapter 5

Warrior II	117	Bear Pose	138
Extended Side Angle	119	Eagle	140
Triangle	121	Standing Leg Raise	142
Humble Warrior	123	Tree Pose	144
Crescent Lunge	124	Dancer	146
Star Pose	127	Balancing Half Moon	148
Wide-Leg Forward Fold	128	Warrior III	150
Big Toe Pose Leg Lifts	130	Standing Splits	151
Pyramid Pose	131	Chair Twist	153
Goddess	132	Crescent Twist	155
Big Toe Pose	134	Seated Twist	157
Gorilla	135	Twisting Triangle	158
Fire Toes Pose	136	Wide Down Dog Twists	160
Yogi Squat	137		

Chapter 6

Locust	176	Headstand	195
Floor Bow	177	Tripod Headstand	197
Reclined Hero Pose	178	Dolphin	199
Camel	179	Forearm Balance	200
Bridge	180	Handstand	202
Wheel	182	Leapfrog Hops	204
Flip Dog	184	Shoulderstand	205
Crow	187	Legs-Up-the-Wall Pose	207
Side Crow	189	Plow Pose	208
Side Plank	190	Fish Pose	209
Forearm Plank	192		

Chapter 7

Frog	223	Lizard	232
Half Pigeon	224	Reverse Tabletop	233
Double Pigeon	226	Seated Forward Fold	235
Cow Face Pose	227	Single-Leg Forward Fold	236
Bound Angle	228	Wide-Angle Forward Fold	237
Half Splits	229	Final Rest	241
Happy Baby	231		

Chapter 8

Boat	248	Plank Curls	251
Scissor Crunches	249	Bicycles	252
Scissor Kicks	250	Crow Crunches	253

FOREWORD

I've been immersed in yoga for my entire life. My parents, Magaña and Walt Baptiste, opened one of the first yoga schools in San Francisco in 1952. They were pioneers in bringing yoga to the West, and many of the teachers they hosted in their school and retreat centers were influential contributors to yoga as we know it today.

When I was a teenager, I had an experience that shifted everything in my life—an experience that completely opened my eyes and heart to live with my purpose and power. I met Mr. B.K.S. Iyengar at a dinner party with my parents, and he invited me to his workshop while he was visiting San Francisco. I knew it was a huge honor to be personally invited by him, but I wasn't very familiar with his style of yoga at the time.

In the workshop with a gymnasium full of Iyengar's dedicated students, I felt like I was in over my head. I had never practiced such an athletic style of yoga asana with such precision and rigor. I suspect Mr. Iyengar sensed me doubting myself when he approached me and requested that I do a drop-back. I didn't know what that was, but I looked around and saw the other students moving from mountain pose to full wheel and back with confidence, strength, and grace. As Mr. Iyengar stood in front of me and asked me to do something I didn't think was possible, something within me shifted in that moment. *I got out of my head and into my body.* I dropped back . . . and came back up. In that moment, I let go of my doubts. I trusted the strength and wisdom of my body as well as the guidance of my teacher. The experience lit a flame within me for the physical practice of yoga.

That one yoga practice sparked a fire within me and set my life in a completely new direction, and it opened me to my life purpose. It led me to develop my own style of yoga, teach yoga trainings all over the world, build an institute committed to training leaders in the practices of yoga and meditation, establish a nonprofit that trains yoga teachers and creates jobs all across Africa and in the United States, and to write five best-selling books. The fiery and physical practice of power yoga is a gateway to so much more than just feeling strong in your body: It's a method for total life transformation of body, mind, and spirit.

A profound physical experience can be a vehicle for changing not only how you see yourself but also how you experience the world. There's an awakening that occurs when you let your mind slow down and let your body lead the way. In a powerful, challenging, and sweaty yoga class, you experience your own strengths and struggles as you challenge your physical and mental limits. Through an intense yoga practice your body reveals the way for you, and you access your inner power. It starts with the physical practice, and the practice illuminates your potential.

Yoga gives you a method to close the gap between what you want, what you know is possible, and who you are. Within every pose, you access and apply your own power through choosing to take action or conscious nonaction, with your inner wisdom leading and the big picture in mind. You decide when to push, when to hold back, and when to let go. Every practice becomes a journey into your own power, and you get to access your power everywhere else in your life—off the mat, where it really counts. The postures are active steps taking you toward how you want to feel, who you want to be, and the life you want to live. The results of your yoga practice are amplified when you learn from a great teacher who will help you on your journey. In this book, Leah will guide you to create a power yoga practice that will enrich and empower your life.

I first met Leah in a yoga teacher training that I was leading on the Big Island of Hawaii. Since then Leah has worked as a part of a core team in my transformational yoga trainings at retreat centers, conference rooms, and yoga studios all over the world. With her clarity and guidance, she has consistently amplified the effectiveness and impact of my trainings and made a real difference in people's lives. Leah is a brilliant teacher and leader, and she masterfully distills the teachings into practical and actionable steps.

In this book, Leah shares how to build a yoga practice that makes a difference for you—one that works for your body, your lifestyle, and your individual goals. She takes the essence of the traditional teachings and adapts them to meet our modern day culture. Through simple steps and short sequences, you'll gain the tools to customize your practice, build physical strength, expand your energy, and harness your power. Leah's instruction will empower you to create your power yoga practice to feel good and fuel your life.

Anyone can do yoga and benefit from yoga; it's a practice that doesn't discriminate. With Leah's expert guidance and this four-week plan, you are sure to build a solid foundation for a lifelong yoga practice. Leah will guide you through the basics, starting with your breath and your reason for practicing yoga. The poses and sequences outlined in this book will help you weave it all together. Trust your body, trust the guidance in this book, and trust the process.

It's been an honor to work with Leah over the years and to see her add her own experience, innovation, and understanding to the practice. I am overjoyed to be a champion for her sharing in this book and to witness her carrying forward the light of these sacred teachings with all of you.

In love and happiness,

Baron Baptiste
New York Times–Bestselling Author
Founder of the Baptiste Institute and Baptiste Foundation
Yoga Luminary and Global Yoga Teacher
Creator of Baptiste Yoga

PREFACE

I found power yoga when I hit a breaking point in my body and my life.

After years of working in the fast-paced world of political campaigns, I allowed my work to consume my life. I was in my mid-twenties when I landed in the emergency room with half of my body going numb.

The numbness had started a few years before with tingling in my right foot when I would work out. I eventually stopped running and doing cardio because the feeling of pins and needles running up my right leg seemed to get worse with movement. After a while, the dull pain had spread throughout my right leg and arm and become a part of my daily life. At the same time, my career was taking off, and I was busy doing the work I had always dreamed of doing. The nagging pain in my body took a back seat to my work and responsibilities.

One morning, after a successful work event, I woke up with my right foot feeling noticeably more asleep than usual. I struggled with putting on my shoe because of the swelling and numbness of my right foot. When I sat down at my desk, I realized that it wasn't just my foot. The loss of feeling and sensation was spreading throughout my whole right side, and it spread through the right half of my face.

I called my doctor, and he told me to immediately go to the emergency room because I was most likely having a stroke. When I arrived at the hospital, the first doctor informed me that, given my age and symptoms, I most likely had multiple sclerosis. I was terrified. In the days that followed, I did my best to work through my flood of emotions, the numerous tests, and the haunting feeling that I could have prevented this if I had been paying attention to my body rather than ignoring signals and working on top of pain, numbness, and trauma that had been building for years.

Back in my first year of college, I was a cheerleader and had a career-ending fall in which I sprained my neck and injured my lower back. I didn't properly rehabilitate my body after my fall; instead, I tried to move on as quickly as I could. At the time, I was working through personal challenges: my parents' difficult divorce, a tough breakup of my own, and feelings of loneliness, confusion, and disappointment. Because of my injuries, I wasn't working out and moving my body the way I was used to. The trauma from my fall got buried, and I did my best to keep pushing forward.

After my trip to the hospital, I went through rounds of tests, tried different medicines, and met with specialists with contrasting ideas of what was wrong with me. It became clear that I needed to take the lead and that it was time to dig deeper. I needed to get back into my body to reconnect to my life.

This humbling experience was my wake-up call. I was stressed out and burned out, and I needed a way back to my power. I recognized that my body was communicating so much more than just nagging and persistent old injuries. I used this breakdown as my opportunity to start living with more purpose and power, and I decided to commit to my practice of power yoga.

Power yoga sparked a whole new way of living for me. It served as my vehicle to rebuild strength, sensation, and connection as I reawakened my body. Rather than doing things the way I had always done them, I started to go within and used yoga as a roadmap for a new journey. In my practice, I was able to get out of my head, and I remembered what it felt like to be at home in my body. My time on the mat became my sanctuary for self-care. I became aware of how, in just a few years of high-stress living, I had literally wound myself into knots. My yoga practice helped me transform and release the heavy energy that had built up inside me from stress, and my attention to my breath helped me feel more calm and centered. Through the yoga poses, breath, and sweat, I started to unwind the knots, and I felt more connected and powerful in my body than I had in years.

Power yoga helped me access my inner wisdom. My daily yoga practice allowed me to listen and respond to the subtle physical messages from my body. (Our bodies are always sending us signals about our health, emotions, thoughts, and well-being and about how to be our most powerful selves. The hairs standing up on your arms, the dull pain in your gut, or the lump in your throat can be your body communicating that something is off or that more is available.) Through my power yoga practice, I started to work with my body, seeing it as my guide and greatest teacher.

As my yoga practice grew, I not only recovered but also became stronger. I didn't realize at the time that my practice would become a vehicle for me to step into my power in all areas of my life. Power yoga is incredibly physical, demands your full presence, and puts you

> Yoga releases the creative potential of life. The light that yoga sheds on life is something special. It is transformative. It does not just change the way we see things; it transforms the person who sees.
>
> B.K.S. Iyengar

deeply in your body. And when you are in your body in the present moment, you can tap into your reservoirs of personal power. With my committed practice, I felt more purposeful in my work, I felt less stressed and more well rested, and I felt more connected and present in my most important relationships. I felt good.

I've experienced this shift myself, and I've seen it unfold with thousands of others. The people drawn to this style of yoga practice often have a sense that something more is available in life but don't know how to get there. With the physicality and mindfulness of power yoga, the body often reveals the way. The body holds wisdom that we're not able to access with the mind. Through vigorous and disciplined work on the yoga mat, I've seen people wake up to depleting habits, patterns of self-sabotage, and unconscious beliefs that have been limiting their freedom and expression for years! After moving through the old energy that had been holding them back, people discover their true desires, articulate their hopes, and start living the life of their dreams.

The more you practice, the more you'll be able to feel. The more you feel, the more receptive you'll be to the message from your body. We call it a yoga practice because it has to be brought to life on an ongoing basis, with commitment and focus. This creates power.

I've experienced the power of yoga firsthand. It started with my physical practice and then expanded into all other areas of my life—into meditation, my way of thinking, my relationships, and the foods I eat. I poured myself into my quest to live a more purposeful and fulfilling life. Through my study of movement, nutrition, and holistic living, I have found a physical and spiritual balance and created daily practices to increase my energy and expand the healing power that I found into all areas of my life. Through it all, I've become lighter, happier, and more free.

I created this book because I believe that power yoga is a pathway to cultivating more energy and vibrancy in our lives today. I am passionate about this practice because of what it has done for my body, mind, and spirit and because I've seen thousands of people use power yoga to transform their bodies and their lives.

This book is designed to help you integrate power yoga into your existing workouts and to give you the tools practice on your own, and the experience to feel more confident in classes, workshops and your daily life. I encourage you to explore the content on your mat, in your relationships, with your work, and in the stillness of your seat in meditation. The more you focus on activating your power yoga practice, the more you will come alive in all areas of your life.

My intention is to share the ancient practices and principles of yoga and wellness and to make them accessible and practical for your life today. Much guidance is available through leaning on the lessons and traditions of those who have come before us. Yoga is a time-tested method that we can use today to create more power, ease, and joy, right now.

I hope that sharing what has worked for me provides guidance for your experience and serves to steer you toward the way that works for you. I love that there is no one way in yoga. Instead, the practice is an invitation for us each to explore and express what feels most true for each of us.

My greatest hope is that you use this book to find your truth as well as personal power and happiness. I hope you share your insights with others to spark connection, peace, and joy and create a positive ripple effect out into the world. Yoga comes to life when we bring it to life.

Now it's your turn. Regardless of what led you here and what sparked your interest in power yoga—whether it is curiosity, a breakdown, or a breakthrough—it is exactly what needed to happen now. Trust that you are precisely where you need to be and that in this book you'll find the tools that you can use right now.

May your practice ignite the power that is within you and light your path forward.

Lokah Samasta Sukhino Bhavantu
May all beings everywhere be happy and free,
and may the thoughts and actions of our lives contribute
to that happiness and to that freedom for all.

ACKNOWLEDGMENTS

I am humbled to be able to share this book and the practice that has transformed my body and my life and, in the process, has opened me to more love, joy, and learning than I ever imagined was possible.

To all of those who contributed to my path to writing this book, my deepest love and gratitude.

Thank you to the following people for their contributions to my life and my work:

My deepest gratitude to all the yogis, sages, and teachers who have walked before me and shared the tradition of yoga.

Thank you to my family for all your love and support.

To my partner, Frankie: You are my rock and my light. Thank you for showing me how to truly be in union with another, and for your unwavering love, honest reflection, and steadfast support. It is my great honor and joy to get to love you and share this life with you.

To my sweet girl, Victoria: Thank you for choosing me. I love you, and I am honored and humbled to be your mama.

To my Mom: Thank you for introducing me to yoga as a teenager and to the world of energy, visualization, and holistic health. I am forever grateful for your sharing these methods and your gifts with me and teaching me how to translate what is felt into content and practices that can be understood.

Deepest gratitude to my teacher and mentor, Baron Baptiste: Thank you for the incredible opportunity to work and study under your wing. Your guidance transformed me as a student and elevated me as a teacher and leader. I am forever grateful for your sharing your genius and your love with me, and for generously contributing the foreword to this book.

To my teacher, Jonny Kest: Thank you for teaching me the roots of the practice and for holding up a mirror for me when I needed it most. You embody the beautiful balance of power and grace.

To Lama Marut: Thank you for sharing with me the philosophical underpinnings of the practice, and for guiding me to live my life as a spiritual practice.

My deepest gratitude for Dr. Wayne Dyer, whose immense body of work has transformed how I think and build alignment in my life.

To Laura Trujillo, my writing coach: Thank you for your guidance and friendship. Your passion and loving encouragement uplifted me and my writing.

Thank you to my soul sisters: Claire Cullis, Jessica Micheletti, Corri Chadwick, Kasee Fuller, and Kate Waitzkin. I wouldn't be the teacher or woman I am today without you all sharing your love, beauty, and grace with me.

To the yoga teachers I have had the honor to learn from and work with over the years, I bow in gratitude. Thank you to my teams at the Baptiste Institute, *Yoga Journal*, and Wanderlust Yoga.

Thank you to the team at Human Kinetics for trusting and believing in me.

Thank you to Jessica Micheletti, Roger Rippy, Gustavo Padron, and Sarah McDonough for contributing your skill, grace, and personal practices to the pages of this book. Thank you Weston Carls for capturing it all. Thank you lululemon, Outdoor Voices, and Manduka for outfitting us. It was a true honor to work with everyone involved in the creation of these photos.

To the many students who I've had the honor to work with in my classes, workshops, and trainings over the years, thank you. I am the teacher that I am because of your allowing me to share this practice and find my voice.

Love and light,

Leah Cullis

INTRODUCTION

It's said that in some major cities there are more yoga studios than there are Starbucks. The 2016 Yoga in America Study (www.yogajournal.com/page/yogainamericastudy) by Yoga Alliance and *Yoga Journal* estimated that over 80 million people would try yoga in 2016, and 36.7 million people consider themselves yoga practitioners. That's up from 20.4 million practitioners in 2012. Yoga is no longer something on the fringe; it's a part of mainstream fitness and wellness, and the benefits are widely embraced. Yoga is working for people everywhere—professional athletes seeking to gain an edge, major corporations aiming to boost productivity and morale, and even parents looking to teach their children the personal empowerment skills that have been left out of traditional education but are necessary to succeed in the modern world. Yoga is a way to focus, feel better, and thrive.

Yoga works for everybody, not just for a few people. I've had the opportunity to work with a range of people —young and old, from elite athletes to those taking their first steps into fitness—and I've watched the magic of yoga open new levels of physical strength and personal power for every single one of them. I've witnessed a transformation on the yoga mat for people from various occupations and walks of life, from business executives to political operatives to homemakers to teens living in townships in South Africa. I've experienced the uplifting shift in my body that happens from just one practice as well as the life-changing benefits that come from a committed power yoga practice, such as relieving daily stress, rehabilitating old injuries, and finding more freedom and peace in my body and in all areas of my life. The one thing that stays consistent through these different experiences is that yoga works. You have to put in the time, commitment, and sweat, but when you do yoga, you will feel the difference. It's so much more than being able to touch your toes or do a headstand. Your power yoga practice will strengthen and support your body, mind, and spirit.

This book honors the traditions and foundations of yoga while demystifying the practices and principles of yoga to make them more inviting, accessible, and applicable for life today. You will access the same benefits as traditional yoga methods while leaving room for adaptation, exploration, and fun.

Why yoga? Because it works.

Power yoga is an athletic, dynamic, and modern style of yoga that is deeply physical and therefore delivers results quickly. In this book, you will learn the poses, practices, and philosophy of this fitness- and focus-boosting method and gain the skills to build a personal practice that creates results that matter to you, both in your body and in your life.

In Sanskrit, *yoga* translates to "yoke," "union," "come together," or "relationship." Yoga is a method for bringing things together. Physically, yoga teaches us how to move in a purposeful and coordinated way. Yoga postures are opportunities to cultivate wholeness in your body so you are not trying too hard in one area or ignoring other parts of your body or who you're being in the process. This practice of moving with your inner rhythm (breath) and skillfully placing your body in a special way (yoga postures) focuses and builds your life force energy—your power.

Yoga is effective because it works with the whole person, not just the component parts. Yoga brings together the body with the breath, the mind with the movement, and the actions with skill. The result is a holistic process that is simple, is accessible to anyone, and has a profound impact on your health, happiness, and heart.

A Brief History of Yoga

Yoga originated in India and was passed down orally from teacher to student. It is estimated to have a 5,000-year-old lineage; the practice predates written history, so the specific time it began is unknown. Yoga first started to make an impact in the United States in the 1950s through a handful of teachers from India. Since then, it has undergone many transformations and adaptations to get where we are today, and it has grown enormously in popularity.

Power yoga emerged in the United States in the 1990s. Baron Baptiste, Beryl Bender Birch, and Bryan Kest all studied traditional styles of yoga and melded their studies with their personal practices as they aimed to make yoga more accessible to a wider audience. They each used the term *power yoga*, which gave each of them the freedom to draw from yoga traditions and poses and create something new. They all kept the physical intensity and athleticism, moved away from a strict sequence, and added their own interpretations and expressions.

The fitness focus and creative new approach to the practice had broad appeal and introduced power yoga into gyms, where people began to see yoga as a workout. Today, you will find power yoga in both yoga studios and gyms across the globe. The heat—the cleansing fire and sweat that comes from a dynamic workout—is the primary ingredient that sets power yoga apart from other styles of yoga. It brings you to your edge, where you challenge your limits.

Yoga is going through a modern renaissance. The benefits from this ancient practice are available in abundance today, and the practices, like power yoga, are designed to meet our modern needs. Although yoga has gained tremendous popularity for its transformative power for the body and mind, it's important to understand where this practice came from. The roots of this life-changing practice are often overshadowed by its immense physical benefits, so let's take a closer look at yoga's origins.

The Eight Limbs of Yoga

The Yoga Sutras of Patanjali is a foundational yogic text written over 1,700 years ago by the sage Patanjali. In it, he outlined 196 sutras, or threads, detailing how to live a yogic life. Patanjali's teachings were mostly focused on meditation. Only a handful of these sutras were about the physical practice, and they didn't include any specific yoga poses, except for a comfortable sitting position. *The Yoga Sutras of Patanjali* is our first introduction to the eight-limb path known as ashtanga yoga. The eight limbs of yoga outline a system for us to follow as we aim to be happier and healthier. In *The Yoga Sutras of Patanjali* we learn that yoga is so much more than a workout; it's a system for optimal living.

The eight-limb path helps you navigate your journey to your inner self. When you look within, you experience and identify with your inner wisdom and spirit. This internal work of personal inquiry reveals your purpose and what's most important to you. Yoga is a system for you to access power that is already there—just waiting for you to unlock, ignite, and share it with the world.

The first two limbs of the eight-limb path are the yamas and niyamas. They are the ethical disciplines of yoga and are often compared to the Ten Commandments—the dos and the don'ts of the practice. The yamas are the ethical restraints, and the niyamas are the moral observances. The guidelines are not meant to limit us but rather to align our daily actions so that life can flow.

Asana is the third limb of yoga and is the physical practice, the yoga poses. Pranayama is the fourth limb and is breath and energy control. The other four limbs—pratyahara, dharana, dhyana, and samadhi—are all levels of meditation. In the West, we often get drawn into the yoga with the physical practice, and there is so much more to this ancient system that is designed to elevate the body, mind, and spirit.

Yamas: The Restraints

Ahimsa: Nonharming
This first teaching shares that we must first do no harm. It encourages us to cultivate the right balance in all relationships so that we are neither harming others or ourselves. In the face of anger or violence, this tenet calls us to be mindful and compassionate.

Satya: Truthfulness
Satya is being honest with yourself and staying true to yourself in your thoughts, speech, actions, and relationships. This goes beyond simply not telling lies. Telling the truth is a pathway to freedom.

Asteya: Nonstealing

Asteya is not taking (or taking credit for) what is not ours and not longing for what others have. This principle reminds us to be mindful of our actions so we are not taking away from others, ourselves, or the planet.

Brahmacharya: Moderation

There's power in moderation. Traditionally, brahmacharya was described as celibacy; through abstinence you could preserve and focus your life force energy. A more modern approach is to be responsible and moderate in how, where, and with whom you spend your energy.

Aparigraha: Nonpossessiveness

Clinging to the material world—people or things—only weighs us down and makes life heavy. This tenet guides us to free ourselves from greed, grasping, and coveting.

Niyamas: The Observances

Saucha: Cleanliness

Saucha calls us to cleanse and purify our bodies and our actions, attitudes, homes, and hearts. When we are free from impurities, we can live with more harmony, clarity, and energy. Let go of the foods, habits, and people that drain you, and align with what feels good.

Santosha: Contentment

Contentment is total acceptance of what is; it is appreciating the moment. Santosha invites us to live in the now and to be grateful for the everyday gifts that are all around us.

Tapas: Austerity

Tapas is the heat that is required for anything to change and grow. It is the self-discipline of developing a new routine, the commitment in a long-term relationship, or the self-control of staying in a challenging yoga pose when your muscles burn and sweat runs down your face. Tapas asks us to trust the process, especially when the heat is turned up.

Svadhyaya: Self-Study

This is the pursuit and daily practice of knowing yourself. If we don't take the time to look within and reflect, we can easily cruise through life on autopilot. Study what drives you, what has shaped you, and how you can be your best now.

Ishvara Pranidhana: Devotion

Devotion is recognizing that we're all in this together and honoring that we are all connected. It is also the trust that something greater is at work. You can trust that the universe has your back and that you are both protected and guided. All you need to do is trust and lean into it.

Asana: Physical Practice

In Sanskrit, *asana* means "seat" or "pose." Yoga poses are opportunities to understand, expand, and explore your energy and power. The practice of asana invites you to honor your body as your temple and learn how to cultivate the balance of effort with ease within you. There's no final destination in any pose; the process of the pose holds the power. Let your body reflect what is true for you.

Pranayama: Energy Control and Breath

Prana translates to "energy," and *yama* means "control." Our energy is circulated through the body on the pathway of the breath. Yogis practice different methods of controlling the breath to increase and expand their energies. Taking a big, deep breath in any moment can shift your energy and put you back in touch with your power.

Pratyahara: Withdrawal of the Senses

This fifth limb reminds us that our greatest power is always within us. When you turn off your awareness to external stimulation, you can start to awaken your inner vision and tune in to your inner wisdom. To be your most powerful self, you've got to tune in to what's going on inside, and pratyahara is the first step on this inner journey.

Dharana: Concentration

Learning to concentrate isn't something that you do once. It's the practice of coming back again and again. Setting your gaze on one point when doing a yoga pose helps you to focus both physically and mentally and, as a result, you start to tune out distractions and tune in to what's essential. Practicing the binding of your mind to an object, place, idea, or practice builds power and focus and prepares you for meditation.

Dhyana: Meditation

When your practice of concentration on a single point of focus is steady and committed, deep meditation and contemplation occur. As you become entirely absorbed in your focus, stress from your body and mind melt away, and you move toward union or bliss. Meditation teaches us the power of presence.

Samadhi: Unification and Oneness

This is the culmination of the practices and the experience of joy and bliss. In this state, you are completely clear of any worldly worries; fully connected to your

The Teachers

These four teachers are credited with having influenced most modern styles of yoga practiced in the West. Many teachers have contributed to the current yoga landscape, but these teachers are the source of many of the teachings.

Tirumalai Krishnamacharya is the yoga pioneer credited with having the most influence on modern yoga. He is responsible for the emphasis on the physical practice, also known as hatha yoga. Krishnamacharya's influence spread yoga across the globe through his three most famous students: Sri K. Pattabhi Jois, B.K.S. Iyengar, and T.K.V. Desikachar.

B.K.S. Iyengar created Iyengar yoga, which focuses on anatomical specificity, precision, and alignment in each posture. Iyengar's book, *Light on Yoga*, was published in 1966 and is still considered one of the most important books for modern yoga.

Sri K. Pattabhi Jois is the father of ashtanga vinyasa yoga, which is a dynamic style that links breath with movement. Ashtanga vinyasa yoga is the primary root practice for power yoga and other modern styles of yoga today. Jois made his first visit to the United States in 1975 to share ashtanga yoga.

T.K.V. Desikachar developed Viniyoga, a method that customizes practices based on the student's unique physical conditions, age, background, and interests and emphasizes yoga's therapeutic benefits.

intentions, body, and heart; and at one with everything in the universe. The ultimate goal of yoga is to be fully liberated and free.

How to Use This Book

This book focuses on how we use the physical practice in the West today and how you can build your power yoga practice. Knowing the foundations of yoga allows you to get the most out of your practice. Leaning on 5,000 years of tradition, power yoga is a challenging physical workout that not only tones your muscles and mind but also strengthens your spirit.

> Power Yoga is about working hard sensitively. It's about feeling good, not just looking good. The tone and shapeliness you attain from this work is a by-product. The focus here is balance and healing.
>
> Bryan Kest

I suggest you start by reading through the whole book. In chapter 2, you will learn about setting your intention. Regardless of whether this is new to you, I recommend setting your intention for your power yoga practice. There is immense power in understanding your why.

Next, read through the whole program to get a sense of all the elements while keeping your intention in mind. Each chapter includes an introduction to why the topic is critical to your yoga life and practice. The chapters will help you learn the basics so you're ready to hit the mat in your 28-day power yoga plan. As you move through the book, if a practice or technique sparks your interest, try it out and start to experiment with what most speaks to you. Once you get to the final chapter, you'll have the foundation you need to get started in your 28-day power yoga plan. In the plan, you can build your custom power yoga practices, and I also provide a master practice to guide you each week.

As you move through the book, you will learn more about the history of yoga, how and why the practice can benefit you now, and how to build a practice that not only feels good but also is sustainable for the rest of your life. Once you are ready to start your plan, each class will begin with an opening pose and sun salutations, move into power poses, progress to optional peak poses for more challenge, and finish with cooling sequences and a final rest. The level of challenge and intensity is up to you, because every practice and every pose are adaptable to meet your unique needs and goals. If you love a sequence, feel free to repeat it and soak up more; if something doesn't work for you, leave it out for now. You get to work the program in a way that serves you and fits your life.

> Yoga is a process of replacing old patterns with new and more appropriate patterns.
>
> Tirumalai Krishnamacharya

To get the most out of your program, commit fully to the 28-day plan. Stay with your power yoga plan for the full 28 days, and I promise that you will see results in your body, your mind, and all areas of your life. Use the book as your resource guide on your journey of this lifelong practice.

Remember that every experience holds a lesson if you choose to look for it. The key to success is making it work for you. The power comes from practice, so let's get started.

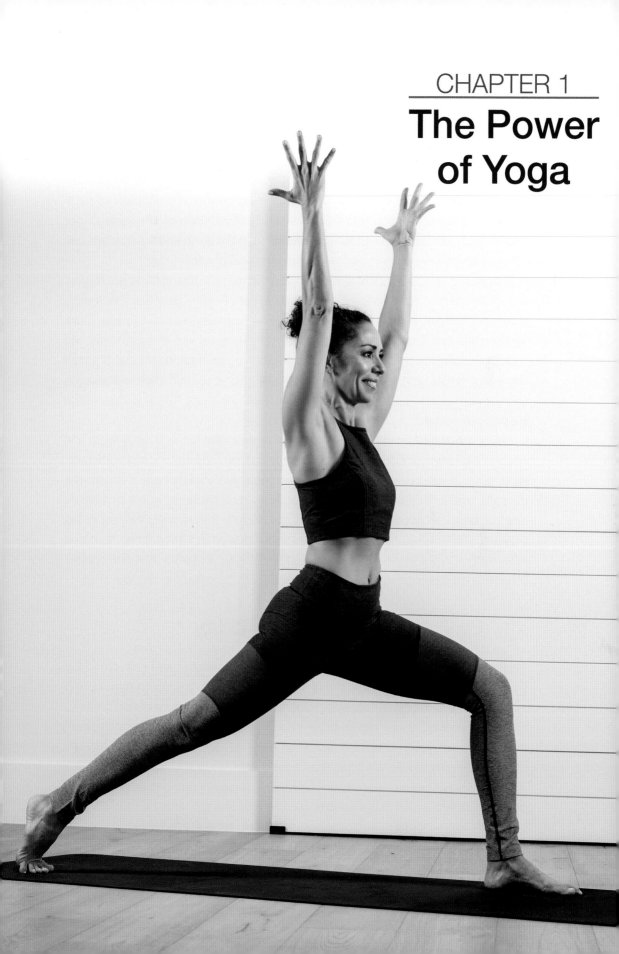

CHAPTER 1

The Power of Yoga

Remember when you felt your most powerful. What were you doing? Whom were you with? What contributed to feeling this way? Whether you were with family, teaching your first yoga class, or achieving a goal you set for yourself, the common thread is that you had this experience. We use empowering and defining moments in life to learn, grow, and help us thrive.

This book focuses on what you felt in those defining moments: the energy of life that comes from feeling good, alive, and fully in your power. The same power runs through all of life and nature—the energy from the earth and the sun. We can connect to this power when we live consciously and purposefully.

Your power is the amount of aliveness you possess. It is the ability to act on your own behalf and to trust yourself and your intuition. Power yoga is an incredibly potent and purposeful method to refine and harness this power within you. It is a practice that raises your vitality and sense of personal power. When you embody your power and are in touch with your strength, you gain confidence and accelerate your results on and off the yoga mat. Power yoga challenges you physically and supports you in building a practice that feels good and helps you create the life that you desire.

Power builds through repetition. In yoga, you create the same shapes again and again to explore your body and measure how you are growing and strengthening. When you cultivate power physically through yoga, you access more of your power mentally, emotionally, and spiritually. As your practice expands, you'll start to see how patterns and habits in your movements and life are working for you, or not working, where you can adapt to increase your power and satisfaction, and how everything on your yoga mat reflects your life. Yoga can be an incredibly potent vehicle when you choose to practice regularly with commitment and devotion.

Yoga for Life Today

While yoga is an ancient practice, power yoga is accessible and relevant today. Our modern lifestyles are full of stress and require us to move fast to keep up. We live in the time of the nonstop news cycle, and answers and information about any topic are just one Google search away. It's said that, on average, American adults check their smartphones around 150 times per day! We are bombarded by stimulation and opinions and are addicted to immediate feedback. Tools that enhance life and increase productivity can also serve as a huge distraction from living in the present moment and with the people who are right in front of us.

In our hyperproductive and overworked culture, we are conditioned to look for "more" on the outside. We look for the next quick fix—the best diet, the right partner, the perfect job, or something to make us feel better. With all this searching, it's easy to feel disconnected from your body and purpose. In the busyness of life today, our bodies get stiff, our minds get restless, and our energy gets stagnant. This way of living is new, inspired by modern technology and advances, but our bodies and spirits still crave the stillness and grounded way in which our ancestors lived and our bodies are designed to thrive.

Yoga teaches us to look for the answers within and awaken from the inside out rather than from the outside in. When you cultivate clarity and power on the inside, you begin to shine your light in all ways. With commitment and focus on this ancient method, you access the results of yoga that are widely known today, all of which means less stress, more energy, and an increased sense of your power to live your life right now. The benefits of a committed yoga practice include the following:

Increased physical strength

Patience

Mental clarity

Connection to self and others

Physical and mental flexibility

Adaptability

Overall health and well-being

> Yoga is not an ancient myth buried in oblivion. It is the most valuable inheritance of the present. It is the essential need of today and the culture of tomorrow.
>
> Swami Satyananda Saraswati

Power Yoga

Power yoga is a fitness-based yoga practice, an American interpretation of ashtanga vinyasa yoga. It has many of the same benefits as the foundational and vigorous traditional practice, including building internal heat and increasing strength, stamina, focus, and flexibility, as well as cultivating meditative breathing and reducing stress.

This potent practice is a complete workout on its own and complements (and offers tremendous benefits when integrated into) other workouts and fitness programs. In addition to strength, power yoga helps develop focus, balance, and purpose within overall fitness and wellness. The precision and pace of the practice help tone and cleanse the entire body, increasing circulation and stimulating lymphatic flow. As you move and lengthen, twist, and fold your body in all directions, you ignite all your major energetic centers and the energetic pathways for your vitality to flow. Detox is fueled with increased breathing, sweating, and stimulating the organs that remove waste and excess from the body. When you shed excess toxins from your body, you can tap into more of the energy and power that is already within you.

By sweating out toxins, burning off extra energy, and releasing neurotransmitters on a very physical level, you clear out the clutter in your body. When you let go of the old, you make space for the new and wake up to what's available right now.

When you lean on ancient wisdom practices like yoga, and adapt them for life today, you can free your energy to trust and be easy on yourself. You don't have to re-create the wheel when it comes to cultivating purpose and energy; you can follow the lessons shared for more than 5,000 years. Look to the teachers and the practitioners who have walked the path before and learn from their trials and errors, breakdowns, and breakthroughs. Simply do the practices and trust the wisdom of the yogis, dedicated students, and teachers who have done the same. Use the time-tested practices within these traditions and apply them to your modern lifestyle, knowing results will come.

Yoga lays out a roadmap for a more fulfilling life today. There is power in being a part of tradition. There is energy in the rituals and repetition of yoga because the lessons are timeless and universal. Power yoga is not about getting it right, achieving, or following one narrow path. It is about applying the ancient system of yoga with the tools available today to make a difference right now, no matter your level or ability.

Trust the practice, trust the tested process, and adapt it to make it work for you.

The Power of Now

The Yoga Sutras of Patanjali is the foundational yogic text written over 1,700 years ago by the yogic sage and philosopher, Patanjali. The text is comprised of 196 sutras, or passages, outlining the foundations of yoga, including the eight-limbed path. The first thread of wisdom he shares is this:

> *Atha yoga anushasanam.*
> Now, the teachings of yoga.

Now is when the practice of yoga begins and where it happens over and over again. We learn right away the importance of *now*—the present moment. This simple statement illuminates the truth that the only time we have power is in the present.

The past has already happened—it's gone and is just memories. The future hasn't happened yet, so it's only thoughts and fantasy about what might happen. The emphasis on *now* in the first passage—in arguably the most important yoga text—is a call for action for us to wake up and live in the now.

The only time and place that we have access to our true power is in each moment as we live it. When we remember this truth, we can use it as an anchor to return into the present moment.

Yoga brings us very deeply into the present moment. Through conscious breath, you get more fully into your body. As you engage physically and intellectually through your senses, you increase the brain's release of dopamine, a neurotransmitter that increases pleasure, motivation, resilience, and perseverance through challenges.

When you are present in your body, you are present for life as it is right now. Yoga practice offers a path to get out of living in your head. When you are living in the now, you can tap into the power and wisdom of your whole body and not just the thoughts in your head. And when you are present, you create space to respond rather than react, choosing to live life in a way that serves your greatest potential. Now is the only time that you have access to this power.

Power yoga is a vehicle for profound change in body, mind, and heart. Only you can do this work, and it can only be done right now. Now is when you can unlock your power and live in the present to discover a more powerful you. Embracing the power of now comes with a beautiful bonus: the freedom to know that everything that got you to right now is exactly what you needed to happen to get to this moment.

That's right. This includes all the struggle, hardships, highs and lows, right and wrong turns, and complete failures of body, mind, and spirit. It was all designed—perfectly—to get you to this place right now. I know it's a bold step to completely trust the path that got you here, and maybe even a bigger leap to trust that you have everything—yes, everything—you need now to move forward. But that's the beauty in this ancient practice. You can lean on the wisdom of the yogis who have come before you, trust the power in the teachings, and try them out in life today. Trust that everything that led you to this moment, this place in your life, this book, and this desire to take on your power yoga practice is exactly the way it's meant to be. Start with the core understanding that everything is whole, perfect, and complete right now; nothing needs to be fixed or changed. You've got everything you need to get started. You don't need to wait until after you get into shape, after you quit your job or find a new one, or

> **Your presence is your power.**
>
> Gabrielle Bernstein

> Start where you
> are. Use what
> you have. Do
> what you can.
>
> Arthur Ashe

after you complete the project you've been working on. It happens right now.

You will build physical strength in your power yoga practice, but you'll gain so much more than that. The power you'll find lies in your capacity to be with and fully present for your life and to live in the now. Even when things get tough and challenges arise, you have the power to be with whatever shows up in your life, exactly as it is right now. It's the power to know that deep down, everything is going to be OK, that you can—and will—get through whatever is on your path. In your power, you can stay and work with what's happening rather than running from it, avoiding it, or numbing yourself. In your power, you can use whatever is happening *for* you.

This may be different from your reality right now, but as you expand your physical and mental strength through this practice, keep this aim in mind, trust this core teaching, and know that this moment is your opportunity to show up as your fullest, most powerful self.

TEACHING TIP
Create a Ritual Before You Teach

Develop your ritual to get clear, present, and grounded in the now before you step into the room to teach. Sharing the teachings of yoga is a great honor, so take time to acknowledge the transition from your busy day to holding space for others. Experiment with designing your ritual for getting present and clear—close your eyes, take a few deep breaths, say a simple prayer, or make an offering before class. I do the same prayer and set an intention before every class I teach. Repetition builds clarity and presence, and being fully present and in the now is the greatest gift you can offer your students. These are some practices for getting present:

- Deep breathing
- Closing your eyes
- Saying a prayer
- Bringing your hands to the heart
- Chanting
- Feeling your feet on the ground
- Touching your head to the earth
- Making an offering
- Setting an intention

Yoga as an Unlearning

It's often said that yoga is more of an unlearning as opposed to something we learn. Yoga leads us back into ourselves and our inner wisdom as we shed the excess, old, and untrue—the energy and beliefs that we naturally pick up through living life today. Therefore, this unlearning is not releasing who you are; it's letting go of all that you are not. In this surrender, you allow your true brilliance and power to shine through.

Yoga works with our bodies exactly as they are, giving us an opportunity to confront and fully be with what's happening. Whatever you experience on the yoga mat is most likely showing up in other areas, so think of your mat as a mirror. The energy of resistance in your body can illuminate some blocks or struggle in another area of life. For example, when we feel unbalanced in life, yoga poses that require you to stand on one foot can feel difficult. When your diet has been heavy and indulgent, twisting poses can feel painful. When you've been glossing over emotions and avoiding issues in your relationships, backbends and heart-opening poses can feel tense and nauseating. The way we practice on the mat is such a great reflection to how we meet life off the mat.

Power yoga brings all the parts of you together for an integrated experience. It's a method for uniting the mind, body, and spirit and teaches you how to breathe, balance, and observe. When you connect what you feel on the mat and what you feel in life, you'll start to notice the moments where you feel the most in tune with your inner strength. You'll start to see where you can edit or adapt your habits or relationships to feel more powerful and purposeful.

> Evolving involves eliminating.
>
> Erykah Badu

The Physical Practice

Traditionally, the physical practice of yoga was designed to prepare you for deeper meditation, connection to a higher source, and spiritual alignment in your life, and this book will explore the potent pathway of the physical practice of power yoga. There are many steps to accessing the benefits of yoga, and ultimately, they all lead to an awakening for a more fulfilling, powerful, and connected life right now. Some choose the pathway of meditation and creating a practice of daily stillness and reflection; some find this inner awakening through artwork and creativity and some through service and devotion to a higher power.

> We are what we repeatedly do. Excellence, then, is not an act but a habit.
>
> Aristotle

Power yoga resets you physically as you clear your body of old and excess energy and generate and invite in new energy. When you practice a physically demanding yoga sequence every day—sweating, breathing, and committing to your body—you will start to transform. There is no question about it. You get out what you put in. The yoga will work on you from the inside out, thus creating a difference. Your diet and habits will change to support the needs of your body and your power yoga practice.

Regular and purposeful movement transforms the energy of your life from an experience that you've had into energy that you can use. If you're not moving, your energy gets stuck and creates blocks or tension in the physical body, which leads to emotional, mental, and spiritual blocks.

The Body

Everything you say, do, eat, and feel leaves an imprint within your body. A stressful conversation can be felt in your chest, neck, and pulse before, during, and after the confrontation. Conversely, an evening of intimate conversation and touch can leave you feeling inspired, connected, and relaxed for days to come. It goes beyond the emotional impact. An evening meal of fresh local veggies and proteins prepared at home will feel very different in your body the next day than a meal of heavy pasta with dairy, meats, and a few glasses of wine. How we live, what we eat, what we think, and how we move creates the energy we experience.

The body is designed to feel and process your experiences and then release them. Often, humans can hold on to old memories and emotions, not just in our brains but in our cells. A common saying in yoga is, "You've got issues in your tissues!" This happens to all of us, but these issues can take on a whole new life if we are not moving our bodies because we spend so much time at our desks, on our computers, and behind the wheel of a car.

When you are not moving your body or are doing repetitive movements, like sitting at a computer every day, old and excess energy starts to flow in the same patterns. These patterns can get stuck inside your tissues and create blockages. Holding on to this stagnant energy over time creates layers that ultimately slow the flow of life force energy, your power, through you. These layers can show as weight gain, muscle atrophy, depression, dull or inflamed skin, fatigue, brain fog, and more.

Over time, these blockages become toxic and can manifest into imbalance, aches and pains, or worse. If warning signals from the body are not addressed, they can quickly escalate into depression, disconnection, injury, and disease.

If you want to feel a different way, then the good news is that the power lies with you to do so. Your body is not static; it responds to your daily actions and what you repeatedly do. What you put into your body, your health, and your daily practices will return to you.

Because yoga is accessible to everyone, health care professionals often prescribe it to help alleviate conditions such as high blood pressure, diabetes, obesity, ADHD, insomnia, autoimmune disorders, and anxiety. These conditions have escalated as we have collectively moved toward a stressful and stationary way of living.

Your body will give you both immediate feedback and progress reports over time about how you are living, what's working and what's not. The body does not lie, so honor your body as your greatest advisor and friend, and the payoff will be big. As you build a trusted relationship with your body, you'll learn how to best support your body and your energy to live your best life now. Update your habits, and you can upgrade your life.

The Body Communicates

Our bodies speak in the language of sensation. This may feel like an intense stretch, pain, tingling, opening, release, or your intuition. In yoga, you can tune in and listen to the communication your body sends you by noticing when and where sensations arise. A regular practice of yoga expands your sensitivity, so you wake up to more sensation, more understanding, and more communication from your body.

Your body will always tell you the truth. It knows what is best for you and holds wisdom that can only be felt. Your body communicates with you all the time, sending you signals and lessons that are uniquely designed for you. In order to listen, you must slow down—in yoga practice and in life—to make space to hear and feel your body. You can listen from the rhythm of your heartbeat, from the pace and depth of your breath, from tightness or freedom in your muscles, from the fluidity of your movements, and so much more.

Think about your life outside of yoga for a minute. When you are speaking with a friend, do you feel heard while that friend is walking on a busy street, returning emails, *and* talking with you all at the same time? Is this when you feel most open to sharing? No! The same goes for the body. To listen to and feel your body, you must honor and care for it. You have to put in the time and invest in creating a connection, just as you would in any relationship. The physical yoga practice empowers you to get into your body and build this connection.

> The journey of a
> thousand miles
> begins with
> one step.
>
> Lao Tzu

Every time you practice power yoga, you put the rest of your life on pause to honor the connection within. Instead of letting your head rule how you live, you can tap into your inner wisdom and listen to the guidance within your body, accessing the power of your whole body and being and not just your brain. Use your individualized signals of sensation, and your inner knowing gives you access to being your most powerful self. Imagine what is available to you when you live from this space, in your full power.

The Sanskrit word *svadhyaya* means "the study of the self." In power yoga, you study from the inside out as you explore the postures of your body and the positions of your mind. As you build your power yoga practice, you will strengthen and transform your body and your mind.

Consistency

The key to success in most any venture is consistency. Practicing power yoga, or any daily routine of health and movement, brings the practice to life. You can read all you want about yoga philosophy and tradition, watch videos online, and read about the benefits of meditation on the many yoga blogs out there today. You can gain a lot of information this way. However, you will only know yoga through your experience. You access the transformational powers of yoga when you do the practice. Simply put, yoga is embodied learning, not informational learning.

In order for power yoga to take root within you, you must get into action and stay in action. Yoga is a practice, a process rather than a race. Through consistent practice, you'll begin to cultivate strength, mental clarity, understanding of self, physical and mental flexibility, adaptability, and vibrancy—all of which means less stress, more ease, and more power in your life right now.

Showing up on your mat to do the same poses over and over requires discipline. The practitioners before us were required to make a huge commitment to the practice and show up daily with rigor and a deep observance to tradition. This is why yoga was very exclusive for centuries and only shared with a select few individuals who would commit fully to the tradition and the sacred path. Today, the opportunity to benefit from this extraordinary practice is widely available. However, we maintain at least one link with early practitioners: To access the results, we must show up, practice, and do the work.

The first part of any new practice can feel awkward. Your yoga practice will require you to rewire both your body and brain. Even if you are an athlete and use your body every day, power yoga is different. How often as an adult do you spend the better part of an hour with your body weight on your hands? A regular practice gives you a daily measure for your growth and needs. Trust that as you repeatedly create the same shapes, your body will start to respond. You will start to find more opening, strength, calm, and inner wisdom within every practice and every pose.

Consistent practice generates and builds energy. You become what you repeatedly do. Through repetition on your yoga mat, you'll start to notice a transformation. When you challenge your body physically every day in yoga, there is no question that you'll feel changes. As a natural result of updating your body through movement, your diet and habits will start to change, helping you live your life in a more powerful way. How you practice starts to filter into the way you relate to everything else in your life. A daily commitment of aligning with how you want to feel and putting this purpose into action eventually becomes who you are rather than what you do. You start to burn brighter on the mat, in your work, with your family, and everywhere else in your life. The key is consistency. The more you do the practice, the more rewards you will reap.

A daily practice can mean something different for everybody. There have been times in my yoga practice when I've been disciplined with my morning traditional ashtanga vinyasa practice, and as a result I gained a ton of physical power in my commitment. Other times the most powerful thing I could do for myself is to step away from my mat and let my body (and sometimes my spirit) heal and rest. Sometimes a block of 20 minutes of sun salutations are all that's available to you in your day; other times, getting to a handful of classes at your local studio each week is possible.

There is no one right way. In this program, you'll explore different pathways as you build your daily practice over four weeks. As you grow your practice, take note of when you feel most powerful and what creates real results for you. You can adapt the concepts and principles of power yoga, and everything in this book, to fit to your life. This power yoga plan will give you the embodied experience of consistent practice. From there, you get to build your practice as it will serve your life. You decide what the results look like for you.

Power yoga is a practice for everybody. All that is required is a desire to grow and your breath. I often

> ## Constant practice alone is the secret of success.
>
> *Hatha Yoga Pradipika*

Commit to Your Studentship

One of my teachers often says, "Teacher and student are two sides of the same coin." To be a great teacher, you must always be a student first. They work together. Your practice of yoga, both on your mat and in your life, develops how you share the practice with others. It's essential to stay in the learning and go to classes and workshops, experience other teachers, and commit to your growth. There is no "end" to yoga, so you'll never arrive in the teacher's seat without being a student—no one will. Yoga is a practice of movement, self-study, and commitment. It is always improving. I firmly believe that to be an effective teacher, I must be committed to my own studentship. And every class is an opportunity to study and serve. The more you study how life, your experiences, and yoga help to shape you and empower yoga, the more you will be able to share the gifts with others.

hear people say that they can't do yoga because they're not flexible enough. However, it's unnecessary to be bendy and fit to start practicing. Yoga poses are opportunities to explore and expand your energy, so you don't have to twist into a pretzel or stand on your head to benefit from this practice.

Results are dynamic because you use your full body and breath and move in a way that nature intended. You activate your muscles, and when your muscles are stronger, you fuel your metabolic fire and burn more fat. Power yoga blends strength building, cardiovascular health, stability, flexibility, focus, and inner peace. It's a practice that brings everything together.

Power yoga is a great entry practice for people looking to get into their bodies for the first time, recommit to their wellness goals, or complement other athletic pursuits. There is a yoga pose for everyone, from elite athletes to those wanting to take their first steps on the path to physical fitness. With hundreds of full-color photos, this book breaks down the poses step-by-step, shares benefits, and offers adaptations to modify and intensify to meet your needs and goals wherever you are in your practice. If you don't have a power yoga practice already, this is an excellent place to start! This book is organized in simple, clear terms so that anyone can benefit from practicing power yoga.

Think of your practice not as a set sequence but as an outline that will give you the freedom and flexibility to work at your level and in alignment with your goals and intentions. Instead of rigid rules, we'll use the roadmaps of the yogis, teachers, and universal laws that have been laid out and studied before us and apply them to life today. Some will fit and some will not, so take what you need and leave what doesn't work to create a practice that works for you. You are the one in the driver's seat.

Power yoga will support you in expanding your health and sense of personal power. There is an opportunity beyond just a workout to access more power through integrating and aligning the body, mind, and spirit within one holistic practice. This practice will challenge you physically and empower you to build habits that feel good and fuel other areas of life.

While the physical benefits of power yoga are plentiful, and alignment and the architecture of the poses are necessary, how we feel in the pose—both how we approach it and how we respond to what comes up for us—is important. One of the aims of yoga is to quiet the mind so that you can be your best in each moment. The physical practice is a doorway into this experience. It offers us the tools to turn our focus inside and explore what we are experiencing and how we can show up as our highest selves in each moment. Power yoga is a practice of purpose and can be a vehicle for creating extraordinary results. The power is in the practice and is the perfect blend of strength, sweat, and spirit.

TIPS TO START YOUR PRACTICE

Preparation is important as you start your power yoga practice. Here are some helpful tips to get you started so that you can get the most of your time on your mat.

- Commit to at least 20 minutes a day. Choose a time when you can consistently practice. An ideal time is first thing in the morning, before you start your day.
- Put your practice on your calendar and do it!
- Find an area free of clutter and as free from distraction as possible. Make sure you have enough space for your mat and to stretch your legs and arms out in all directions.
- Invest in tools to support your practice, such as a nonslip mat, two blocks, and a strap.
- Turn off your phone during your practice.
- Avoid eating two hours before you practice. Practice is best on a relatively empty stomach to support your work of deep twists, inversions, and core work.
- Make sure you hydrate, especially after your practice.
- Wear fitted clothing that won't catch or get in the way of your practice. You'll spend a lot of time on your hands, so fitted shirts are best to support you while you sweat and so clothes don't fall over your face and constrict your breath.
- Flexibility is not required. The poses are more about how you feel rather than how you look.
- Have fun. A light heart and open mind are important for this lifelong practice.

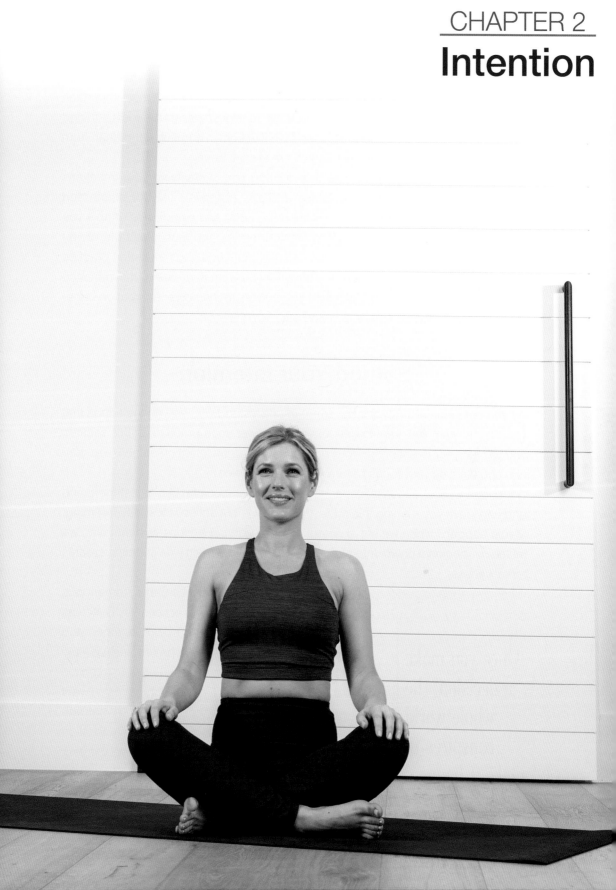

We live in a fast-paced world hyperfocused on outward results, promotion, and success. Constantly looking outward and to others disconnects you from what matters most: your connection to yourself, your power, and your spirit.

Yoga, meditation, and setting clear intentions plug you into what's most important. When you create inner alignment, your actions, relationships, and words are fueled by your inner guidance system. You can then live from inspiration rather than from an outer influence or by the way things have always been.

This chapter explores practices that support you in clarifying your intentions and cultivating focus. When you infuse a bigger purpose into your breath and movements on the yoga mat, you create the energy and experience of how you want to feel. You will have this energy in your bones and musculature, and you can tap into it whenever you want. You can use your yoga and meditation practice as a training ground, your laboratory for what you want to create and experience everywhere in your life. Intention gives you access to the power of creation rather than repeating what is familiar or automatic.

Setting Your Intention

As you begin this journey, it's important to understand why you do the things that you do and what you want to get out of your power yoga practice. In this section, you will set your intention for your program. Setting an intention establishes your aim and clarifies your focus before you get into action.

An idea without action is just an idea. Action without intention is just the doing and can leave you running in circles. Intention without action is just daydreaming. Magic happens when we set an intention and align our actions with that aim; we infuse our personal power into each step on the path. Action with intention creates effectiveness.

> Once you make a decision, the whole world conspires to make it happen.
>
> Ralph Waldo Emerson

The work of Dr. Wayne Dyer has had a tremendous impact on my life and personal practices. Dr. Dyer was the great American philosopher, author, teacher, and pioneer in the fields of self-development and spiritual growth. He would often share that setting your intention is like thinking from the end. First, identify what you want and see it clearly. When you identify what you want, you can use every experience as an opportunity to align with and create what is most important to you. If your intention for your power yoga practice is to feel more freedom in your body, then every interaction—both on and off your mat—can become an opportunity to feel more freedom in your movements, thoughts, or relationships. It's the same energy, and it's all felt. This way of operating takes a leap of faith, but the more you identify what you want, the more you will begin to create it.

In the tradition of yoga, *sankalpa* is the practice of realizing the desires of your heart and moving forward to achieve your highest aim. *Sankalpa* means "wish" or "intention" and joins the mind, heart, and body to create results that align at your deepest level of being. As you honor this desire with your actions, it's said that you not only uncover but also begin to live your *dharma* or divine life purpose. Sankalpa provides a focus for your yoga practice, and connects you to a higher vision for your life. Your intention keeps you rooted in purpose and connected to your power.

Align With Your Higher Vision

We can feel stuck or disconnected from our power because we haven't created a clear vision of what we want. It's easy to get caught up in the day-to-day doing of life without pausing to reflect on what you really want and how you want to feel. This disconnection or lack of a higher vision, a higher aim, can easily lead to feeling uncertain about what you're working toward and like you are just going through the motions. This can leave you feeling stuck, alone, overwhelmed, anxious, uninterested, or like you want things to be another way but aren't sure how or why.

A higher vision leads you to the next steps and lights the way on your path. It helps you decide where it's important to focus. Think of it as a clarifying tool: It helps you align with what fuels you and feels good and steers you away from what depletes your energy. A higher vision, your intention, allows you to move with purpose and power, whether it's on your yoga mat, in your career, or how you relate to the clerk at your local store or with your family. This means rewiring of your brain as you choose to practice looking for the higher good and what unites us. Look to your higher vision; realign and reintegrate with every step.

Let your intention be your guide as you read through this book and every time you step onto your mat. The reflection work will help you peel back the layers and clarify your purpose. When you start to wander or wonder, refocus on your intention for your next step and realign with the energy you want to feel. When you infuse your intention into your actions, everything you do becomes an opportunity to purposefully move in the direction you want to go. Setting your clear aim empowers you to live less out of habit and more from intent.

> Be the change you wish to see in the world.
>
> Gandhi

> The power of intention is the power to manifest, to create, to live a life of unlimited abundance, and to attract into your life the right people at the right moments.
>
> Dr. Wayne Dyer

Guide Your Intention Through Reflection

Take out a piece of paper or your journal and something to write with and answer these open-ended questions to find your intention for your power yoga practice. As you clearly see the results that you want to create, you align yourself with the energy to support your desires.

Let your intention be your guiding light as you deepen your power yoga practice. As you read through this book, periodically review your answers. Focus on your intention, be in the practice of aligning with your higher vision and use your answers as guidance on your path.

Consider the following questions in your life right now:

Where in your life do you feel you are fully present?

Where do you feel most powerful?

What are your daily habits that support you in feeling your best?

How do you want your power yoga practice to support you in your life?

How do you want to feel when you wake up in the morning?

How do you want to feel in the middle of your day?

How do you want to feel when you go to bed at night?

Whom do you want to spend more time with?

What in your daily life feels depleting or draining?

Where do you have a sense that something more is available?

Where in your life or relationships are you lacking focus or direction?

Where have you been holding back?

Where are you stuck?

What do you stand for?

How do you want your power yoga practice to support you in your life?

What do you want to get out of your experience with this book?

Take a moment to reflect on your answers. What stands out to you? Do you see any themes? Reflection work and journaling can help reveal unconscious or limiting patterns and habits as well as deep desires and areas of untapped energy. When you shine the light of your awareness on what is pulling at your attention or draining your energy—and conversely to what your heart and spirit are calling for more of—you can begin to take purposeful action and live in greater alignment with your higher calling. Simple shifts in how you show up daily can create a massive change for your body, mind, and spirit.

Set Your Intention Through Meditation

This physical practice of yoga (asana) is classically designed to be preparation for meditation. The yoga postures were, and still are, used to release excess energy to calm the mind and soothe the nervous system. As a result, you can more easily sit in stillness for meditation. In the simplest terms, meditation is being quiet and going within. It's taking a moment to pause, tune in, and return to your center. It can be as simple as taking a mindful, deep breath to clear your mind and refresh your thinking.

The benefits of meditation have been known for thousands for years and are practiced in traditions all over the globe. It's becoming increasingly mainstream: Everyone from CEOs to elementary school children experience the life-changing effects of meditation. With meditation, you can train your brain to respond differently to stress by practicing being still and focusing on quieting your mind. The mind will run and thoughts will try to pull you away, but the more you return to your single focus, like your natural breath or intention, the more you train the mind to be still and calm. When you build this muscle memory, you can tap into it anytime, especially when you are feeling challenged.

Meditation is a tool for stepping out of distraction and into direction. In the stillness of meditation, the noise and chatter of life is quieted while you take a break from "busyness" of technology, stimulation, and the constant pull of thoughts in your active mind. In slowing down and consciously creating a pause, you tap into what is unchanging within you: your center, your spirit, your power. To prepare for meditation, follow these steps:

> Yoga is the cessation of the fluctuations of the mind.
>
> *The Yoga Sutras of Patanjali:* Yoga Sutra 1:2

❶ Grab a block and create your seat for meditation. Sit on the block at its widest so that you support both sit bones. You can always add more props, such as another block, blankets, or a cushion to make it comfortable so you feel supported. I recommend sitting in one of two positions—sukhasana, which is a crossed-leg position (see figure 2.1a) or virasana, which is a kneeling position (see figure 2.1b). Choose the position that feels best for you.

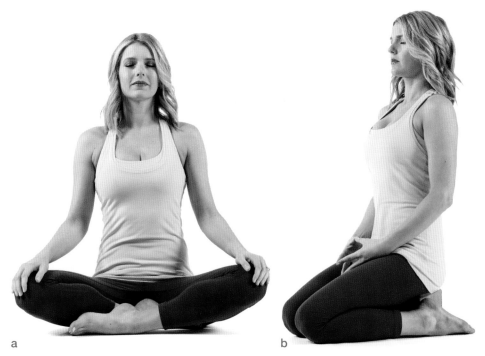

a   b

Figure 2.1   Meditation positions: *(a)* crossed legs and *(b)* kneeling.

❷ Anchor your sit bones down and let the lower half of your body become heavy. Set your hands on your legs, placing your palms down is more calming, and placing your palms up is more energizing. If you prefer another hand position (mudra), feel free to use that instead. I like to connect my fingertips and place my hands in my lap. Next, reach the crown of your head high and sit tall. Close your eyes.

❸ Take three deep breaths in through your nose and out through your mouth to settle into your body. Seal your lips and bring your awareness to the natural flow of your breath. Create a peaceful rhythm with your breath, inhaling and exhaling through your nose, and smooth out any rough edges between the transitions from your inhales to your exhales with each cycle of breath.

4 Shift your awareness to the base of your spine. Now, follow the line of your spine up along your back to the crown of your head. Notice the space and the energetic quality of your spine. This is the place of connection within your body, uniting your right and left sides. Keeping aware of your spine, your centerline, zoom out and get a sense of your entire body, up to the barrier of your skin. Notice how your body feels from your center outward. Notice any tightness and constriction, or relaxation and ease, within your body. Look for patterns of holding stress and areas of freedom. Take 10 breaths or more to explore and investigate the energy within your body as you sit in stillness.

5 Pull your awareness back to your center and settle your attention to the space between the eyebrows. This is your third eye, a major energetic center. Notice any sensation that arises as you lift your attention to this point. Where your mind goes, energy flows. Check in with your breath.

6 Drop your awareness down into your chest, your heart center. Notice the quality of energy in the center of your chest and how the structure of your body forms around this major energetic center. Listening from this place within your body, Ask yourself the following questions:

> What brought you to your power yoga practice?
>
> What do you want to create as you begin your practice and invite more power into your body?
>
> How will you use this new level of power in your life?
>
> We all come to yoga seeking something more. Something bigger is available to us: more love, connection, flexibility, ease, satisfaction. What do you sense is available for you? Expand your awareness out from your body and look into the areas of your life. Ask yourself the following questions:
>
> How do you want to feel?
>
> How do you want to feel in your work?
>
> How do you want to feel with your loved ones?
>
> How do you want to feel when it's just you?
>
> What do you want others to feel when they are in your presence?

7 Listen from the center of your chest and your inner wisdom. Look for the themes in your answers and begin to connect the dots. Can you boil these feelings, these intentions, these energies down into one word that encompasses all that you want to feel? Stay in stillness and listen until you hear a response from within. When you have your one-word answer, lift your prayer

hands to meet at your heart center (anjali mudra). Repeat your word, this energy, to yourself three times. What does it feel like in your body when you focus your mind on this energy, your one word? How does it resonate within you?

8 This word that you uncovered through your inquiry can serve as your intention, or the start of your intention, for your power yoga practice. It can serve as your intention every time you step onto the mat. With this intention fueling your actions, you will create real results that matter to you, both on and off the mat.

9 To finish, bow your chin to chest and release your palms to thighs. Blink your eyes open and lift your gaze. Congratulations on meditating!

Cultivating Focus

Drishti is Sanskrit for "focus." Your focus is essential to establishing your power on the mat. Drishti is your physical gaze, and it's also your intention or focus for your practice.

Physically, when you gaze at one point, you can start to calm your nervous system, hone in on what's essential in the moment, and awaken your insight from the inside. This allows you to tune in to your inner guidance rather than being distracted by the stimulation happening around you all the time.

The quality and energy of your gaze is important. Be clear about what you're focusing on, without being fixed and rigid around your vision. Focus on one spot that doesn't move, then begin to soften your gaze around your focal point. Remain aware of the periphery so you can be open and receptive to the bigger picture, life, and the people with you. As you create stability with your vision, you start to embody stability physically.

> Yoga is the journey of the self, through the self, to the self.
>
> *The Bhagavad Gita*

Energetically, a focus or drishti gives you an opportunity to align with your why every time you step onto your mat. Every pose can be a chance to fuel your purpose within your practice. This happens by putting your attention on what you want to have happen. It holds true in your power yoga practice, your teaching, and everywhere in life.

Yoga and the practice of drishti teaches you to take your attention off what's not going your way and what you want to change. Focusing on what isn't working in

If you ever feel lost or disconnected from your intention, take 30 seconds to realign with your intention. You can do this anywhere!

1. Close your eyes, take a big breath in, and fill up. Then open your mouth, exhale, and clear your body with your breath.

2. With your eyes closed and your breath moving, bring your awareness to your heart center and ask yourself how you want to feel.

3. Lift your shoulders to your ears, then roll your shoulders to your back and open across your chest.

4. Align your body to open to your power. Let your body (your asana) reflect your intention to embody your power.

5. Sit or stand tall, with an open chest. Now ask the question again: How do I want to feel?

6. When you hear your answer, open your eyes and move forward with clarity and purpose.

a situation simply expands and empowers what's not working. Your energy and attention go there, and the result is that you get more of what you don't want.

In a yoga pose, if you are constantly focused on what your body can't do, how the person on the mat in front of you is doing something that your body will never do, or what doesn't feel good in a pose, your practice can feel narrow and draining. Focusing on limitations is depleting and depressing; there is no power in staying focused on what's not working.

Instead, look to the opportunity. Shift your vision to what's working, what you want to have happen, and where you want to go. When you look for how a yoga pose can feel good for you, the overall energy of your experience, where you can access the most breath, and how to create a balance of both effort and ease, the same yoga pose can be a completely different experience. It's not the pose that matters; it's the energy you focus on and create within it. When you look for the opportunity, you make a life-affirming, high-vibrational choice, and you choose more energy. You choose to be powerful.

Setting your drishti is looking for where there is energy and where you can access your power—simply put, you are looking for the light. There is always opportunity to see things in a way that serves you rather than limits you. When you shift your vision to what you want to happen,

> The only thing that can grow is that which you give energy to.
>
> Ralph Waldo Emerson

This simple exercise illustrates the power of your physical gaze and how it affects your overall focus. Notice when you feel most powerful and how you feel physically and mentally when you start to lose your focus.

1. In a comfortable seat, bring your hands to your heart center and shift your gaze to your fingertips (see figure 2.2*a*).

2. Focus only on the curves of your fingers and the connection of your palms. As you keep your focus on this one point, also become aware of what's in your periphery. Notice the floor beyond your prayer hands, the outline of your legs, the color of your clothing. Stay focused on your fingertips. Notice that your focus on one point creates awareness of all points.

3. Keep looking at your fingertips and slowly start to move your hands apart to a few inches between your palms (see figure 2.2*b*).

4. Maintain your focus, your drishti, on your fingertips. Notice in your field of vision the floor between your hands starts to come into your view, but still focus on your fingertips.

5. Now slowly widen your hands even further apart.

6. Stop when you lose your drishti of your two fingertips. You've gone too far—your focus has become too broad—and you have lost your drishti.

7. Slowly bring your hands back together and look at your fingertips. Regain your focus. Pause when your hands are a couple of inches apart.

8. Feel the energy, the tension, between your palms. Move through that energy as you reseal your prayer hands and look to your fingertips.

9. Take three deep breaths with your hands back at heart center, anjali mudra.

10. Gently release your hands to your thighs and lift your gaze.

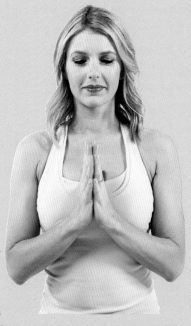
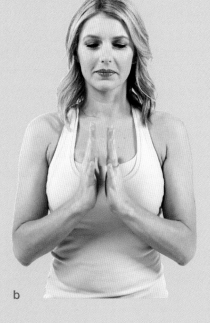

a

b

Figure 2.2 Drishti hand placements.

how you want to feel, and what you can do, you empower these thoughts, actions, and energies for yourself and others. Where your mind goes, your energy flows.

Off the mat, drishti is your higher vision. It means setting your goal as a yogi and incorporating that intention into everything you do, on and off the mat. If you ever feel lost or like you've strayed in your practice, pause and return to your intention and your drishti. Drishti helps us to stay focused on the possibility.

After practicing the exercise described in the sidebar on page 24, you now you have the experience of setting and losing your drishti or gaze. That exercise is the same off the mat. When you try to do too much, everything becomes blurry. Things get mixed up, your body responds by jumping back and forth between multiple points of focus, and you can literally lose your balance. Too much space can lead to disorganization or feeling frazzled or overwhelmed. When you feel like this on and off the mat, use drishti to reestablish purpose. Set your gaze to a stable point. Once your focus is set, start to build your pose from the ground up to embody more stability, balance, and calm.

There is energy and power in seeing clearly both what is in front of you and what you want to create in your practice and your life. Access your power by focusing your attention on what you want and weaving that through all that you do.

Turn Your Attention Inward

Yoga practice gives us an opportunity to study life from the inside, rather than constantly reacting to what's happening on the outside. When you step onto the yoga mat, you can put the rest of your life on the shelf. This pause in commitments and stimulation can offer huge rewards. It creates an opportunity to turn your focus inward. When else do you let yourself entirely unplug from what's happening around you and tune in to what's happening within you?

The fifth limb of the eight-limb path of yoga is pratyahara, which means withdrawing your external senses from outside stimuli by directing your attention internally. This allows you to step back into yourself and objectively observe what is going on within, without the distractions of the world moving around you. When you shut off your external focus, you awaken your inner vision. Put your phone away, tune in to your breath, and let your body guide you into deeper understanding and awareness. When you look within, you will be guided to new levels of purpose, wisdom, and power.

As you move through this book and build your practice, check in with your intention and realign with your higher vision as needed. The practice of drishti, just like every pose, isn't about performing perfectly. It's about taking action that feels true to you at the heart level in every moment and beginning again when

> In order to carry a positive action we must develop here a positive vision.
>
> Dalai Lama

you fall or wander. Every time you come to your mat, you will be united with the bigger intention behind your physical practice that will help you accelerate your efforts. Your intention, your higher vision, makes your practice mindful and not just physical. When you understand your what and why, the how becomes easy and natural.

Applying the Right Effort

Every part of your power yoga practice follows this wisdom: Be clear in your aim and apply the right amount of effort to achieve your desired results. In your power yoga practice, you strengthen physically and emotionally and build your energetic reserves by choosing how hard you're willing to work in each moment. You can choose to stay in a pose as your muscles shake or to rest. You can choose to resist the discomfort or to soften into it. You get to decide what challenge or adversity looks like for you.

PRACTICE GRATITUDE

Gratitude is acknowledging, appreciating, and aligning with all that is good and going well in your life. It's one of the fastest ways to put your drishti into action, which leads to more of what you want. By choosing to focus on all the good in your life in your first waking moments with this simple practice, you will start your day feeling centered, appreciative, and focused on the positive. Before you get out of bed in the morning is a great time to practice gratitude because you start the day by aligning with your best intentions before your feet even touch the floor. The steps that follow will help you accomplish this.

1. In the first moments that you are awake, keep your eyes closed and take a few deep breaths. Ask yourself, What am I grateful for today?

2. Make a mental list (or a written or verbal list) of all the things you are thankful for, listing as many as you can to express your gratitude. Put your focus on everything that is going well!

3. When you come to a natural stopping point, say one more thank-you. Open your eyes, set your feet on the earth, and begin your day grounded in gratitude.

When you express gratitude for the people and blessings in your life, you invite more of the same. Look for the opportunities, big and small, to express gratitude and make it part of your daily practice.

If you are not clear about your aim and the effort you put into your practice, yoga can quickly become just another task to check off on your list. In every breath, you can look within and approach your practice in the way that best serves you now. The continuous infusion of your higher intention into your practice creates a mindfulness in action. Your intention, your high-vibrational thoughts, and your choice to look for the good are some of your greatest tools in accessing your power—and they are available to you at any time through a shift of your focus.

> When you change the way you look at things, the things you look at change.
>
> Dr. Wayne Dyer

Make It Your Own

We all have intentions behind why we practice power yoga, and on the yoga mat, we all work with different sensations, challenges, and strengths. Your whole life contributes to how you feel in your body now, so each yoga pose you create will be a combination of your habits, how your bones are shaped, how active you are, the thoughts you think, and so much more!

As you align with your aim for your practice and apply the right energy in each pose, it's important to remember that there is no one way to create a pose. You've got to make it your own. All yoga poses are opportunities to explore and expand your energy. Every pose is adaptable and can either modified down or intensified.

Nobody is the same, no life is the same, no yoga practice is the same. Alignment principles and practices help inform your activation and focus within the poses for more power and energy. This means that in power yoga, we can take out "doing it right" or "wrong" and go for what is healthiest for your body. I've found the most power in my own practice and witnessed my students break through into whole new realms of experience when we go for what feels good, the greatest expression.

Let Go of Perfectionism

Teaching and leading others takes courage and skill. When you teach power yoga classes, the aim is to help students generate and expand their life force energies and their senses of what is possible in their bodies and lives. These are big goals! If you're using your energy in class worrying about messing up, saying the wrong thing, or forgetting your sequence, you're focusing on you rather than your students. Free your energy so that you can fully be with for everyone that showed up for your class. Let go of trying to be perfect. I've taught a lot of classes, and I've messed up, said the wrong thing, cued the wrong side, or had an awkward moment in every single one of them, and sometimes I've completely fallen flat for an entire class. Teaching is a practice, just like asana. Sometimes you'll go through the motions, other times you'll nail a pose that you've been working on for a long time, and other days you'll completely surprise yourself and learn so much in the process. The thing with both teaching and practicing is that you have to keep showing up and know that falling and picking yourself back up is all part of the process. Some days you'll stumble, and some days you'll shine. The more you let go of your ideas of right or wrong, and let go of trying to be perfect, the more you can learn in every class, connect with your students, and allow your creativity and clarity to develop in your teaching. Plus, when you allow yourself the freedom to be imperfect, you give your students the permission to do the same. Let go of the worry and have fun!

We can look at two different people doing the same pose, and the experience, sensation and satisfaction will be different for each. Take eagle pose (garudasana), for example. Many of the traditional yoga books and teachers tell you to wrap the lifted foot behind the standing leg. That is an excellent goal, but it doesn't work in my body. I have muscular legs from years of sports and lots of scar tissue in my ankles from multiple sprains on the basketball court and soccer fields. Occasionally, I can get the wrap of my foot, but when I do, my whole pose and all the sensation I feel becomes about the position of my lower legs and feet. My whole torso shifts, my breath tightens, and I wince as I go for the pose the way it looks in the book. When I do this, my experience is narrow, out of balance, and painful.

However, I've learned that my greatest expression in eagle is to adapt the shape to meet the unique needs and shape of my body. I use the general shape of eagle as a guide. I press down through my standing foot to get grounded, wrap my legs together, and hug to my centerline, and I deliberately place my toes to the outside of my standing leg for stability. From there, I can get deeper in subtle ways that are unique to me each time I step onto the mat. I can deepen my breath, I can align my shoulders over my hips, and I feel a sense of ease that's not possible when I attempt to mirror someone else. This adaptation gives me access to a more holistic experience, which is the aim of yoga.

I could give you all the alignment cues that I've studied about eagle, but they don't necessarily apply to you. I could tell you how a pose should look and feel, but then you will be searching for a destination based on someone else's experience. That's limiting. Or, I can share general principles of alignment so you can apply them and decide if the sensation or results are serving you.

I can give you guidance to bring to life the general shape and intention of the pose within your body, and you get to discover your practice within that. This is embodied learning rather than informational learning. Use the yoga poses to connect to and create how you want to feel, rather than coming from *this* is the way to do asana. After all, it's all an experiment, and everything is adaptable. The poses are opportunities for you to explore where you are most powerful, rather than getting it right. Find what fits for you from the inside and create the outer form, your expression.

Find Your Edge

On the yoga mat, you're inviting stress and discomfort by putting your body in a series of challenging poses. You learn to stand on one foot and wrap your arms into a bind, hold a lunge for several minutes, and expand your chest and arms while twisting into new shapes. It may not be easy or comfortable at first, but you can learn to do it with breath and ease. In experiencing and confronting discomfort on the mat, you can train your brain and your body to be at ease when stress comes to you off the mat; thus, you can build a relationship to stress that comes from choice rather than reaction.

Your edge is your space of growth. It's the sweet spot for you, the place between too much and not enough, and your unique edge changes every time you practice on the mat—it evolves as you do. You must step out beyond your comfort zone and your habits to get there.

However, your edge isn't about forcing or making something happen. This can feel counterintuitive for many type A personalities who are drawn to the deeply physical style of power yoga. But sometimes we have to slow things down or back things up to allow for growth. It's important to remember the yogic principle of ahimsa or nonharming. It asks us to look at how we are practicing and who we are on the mat. Are we constantly hurting ourselves in postures and always pushing our limits? Too much strength and too much pushing can create more of what we don't want: overexertion, overstimulation, injury, and stress. Stepping up to your edge, yet not beyond it, is a key element of power yoga.

For some, this edge will be flexibility; for others, the edge will be building strength. Sometimes your edge can show up in simply staying in the heat when the going gets tough. When you feel resistance start to arise—physically or mentally—this is a signal from your body and brain that you are near your edge or your perceived limit. It is time to lean in and listen to your inner guidance, align with your higher aim, and apply the right effort. This is where the magic happens.

CHAPTER 3

Power Principles

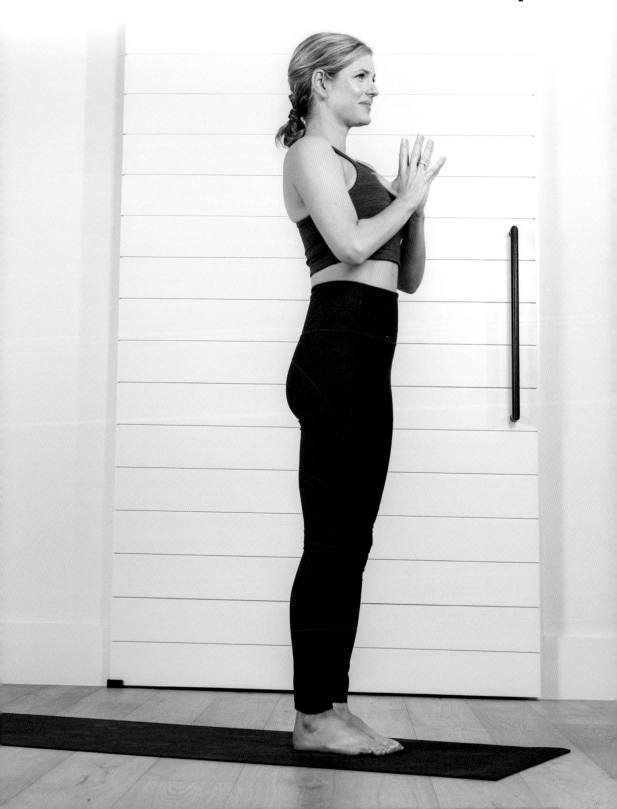

This chapter will explore the principles of building power and the underlying philosophy of the power yoga practice. We'll break down yogic breath, the foundations and actions of all poses, the cleansing internal heat that we build during practice, and linking breath with movement. These principles are the essence of this ancient practice. When you infuse them into your practice, you elevate your workout into a transformational experience.

Breath

Breathing is automatic and happens all day long without you having to pay attention, making it the most basic function of human life. We can survive days without food and water, but only a few moments without breath. Breath gives life.

Yoga creates an awareness of your breath and brings a consciousness to your breathing. Breath is the biggest tool to ignite your personal power on and off the mat. The more you breathe, the more you reap the following benefits:

Increased immunity

Emotional calmness and relaxation

Improved respiration, circulation, and digestion

Relief from physical tension and stress

Accessing suppressed feelings and emotions

Clearing the body of old, stale, and excess energy

Creating a bridge between body and mind

Power yoga is a breath-centered practice, so you move at the pace of your breath. This method combines physical poses and transitions linked with breath to create an extremely effective practice. We either coordinate one breath per movement or hold poses for five breaths or more. If linking breath with movement is new to you, it will take some practice. But once you get there, your breath becomes your guide in your power yoga practice. Like everything in nature, in power yoga, we move with a beautiful, purposeful rhythm.

> The breath is the key to unlocking your body's potential.
>
> Baron Baptiste

Quality of Breath

The way you breathe profoundly affects your quality of life. Your breath reflects the quality of your inner energy and your nervous system. When you are stressed, your breath can get choppy and short. If your breathing is shallow, it likely involves your upper lungs and uses only a small percentage of your capacity and deprives your body of oxygen, energy, and power. When you are at ease, your breath is calm and balanced. There is power in tuning into the quality of your breath, noticing the feedback from your body and your inner energy and letting it guide you from the inside out.

> Anybody can breathe. Therefore, anybody can practice yoga.
>
> T.K.V. Desikachar

When you establish breath control, you also control the fluctuations of the mind. In chapter 2, we looked to the guidance of the second yoga sutra and learned that yoga and meditation calm the mind. By tuning into the quality of your breath and the sensations of your body, you can begin to distinguish your physical form from the thoughts running through your mind—and understand that you are not your thoughts. When you calm the chatter of your mind, you can listen to your body's cues and your intuition. You can make choices and take action that come from insight and understanding rather than from raw reaction and emotion. In every moment, your breath holds valuable information that is uniquely designed for you, where your mind, body, and spirit work as one. The breath is the thread tying it all together.

You can use your breath to feel more calm, centered, and focused anytime you experience intense emotion or the spike of adrenaline, like before a big presentation, race, or game. Simply pause and take a few deep breaths to access your center, where you are the most grounded and powerful. Many athletes have their own rituals to be powerful in their bodies, and often these rituals include turning inward and taking a few deep breaths. What would happen if you incorporated this into not only your game-day ritual but also your workouts or daily routines?

Breath creates presence. When you are aware of your breath, you automatically become aware of your body. Breath is your anchor for awareness and creates a bridge from the outside world to what's happening inside. When you are in tune with your body, you can be present for life as it is right now. You access the power and wisdom of your whole body, not just the thoughts in your head. Let your breath absorb the distractions and fuel your presence.

The breath is your body's gauge during asana practice. If you notice that your breath is getting lazy or automatic, that's your body's cue to bring more attention or power to each breath. If your breath is labored or stressed, that's a cue from within to take it easy or go into child's pose—to come out of the flow and back into your center. Notice when your mind wanders during your yoga practice and use the sound and sensation of your breath to return to your body and what you're doing right now. You can ignite this connection and train your body and mind to cocreate with your breath in your power yoga practice.

In my previous career, I worked on political campaigns and slept next to my smartphone. I was constantly living life in my head—I always had an eye on political blogs, the 24-hour news cycle, and what was happening outside of me. When I started practicing power yoga, which is so deeply physical, it required me to stay connected to my breath to stay in my body and the present moment. This shift to actively incorporating breath was the key to changing my whole world! It set me on the path to being fueled by my inner guidance rather than external stimulation and demands—my breath led me to my power.

There are many techniques for working with the breath. This book will focus mostly on ujjayi pranayama. *Ujjayi* is commonly translated to mean "victorious breath." This breath builds a transformative heat from the inside; energizes the body by oxygenating the blood; and creates a deep, rhythmic sound that provides a focus for the mind and body. The sidebar on page 35 shows you how to use ujjayi breath.

Expansion and Contraction

In power yoga, we match each breath with purposeful movement, amplifying the opportunity to cleanse your body and renew your energy. With each breath cycle, you create physical expansion and contraction, awakening the entire body. The breath creates the pathway for your body to move.

Exhaling empties the old air, clearing out stagnation, toxins, and tension throughout the body. With each exhale, you draw from your physical periphery into your center, your core. As you empty your body of air, you rinse out and create space for something new as you prepare for the next deep breath in.

Inhaling creates space as you stretch from the inside out and fully engage your whole form. The breath opens and expands from your physical center out in all directions. You bring in new, fresh life force into your body and brain. The inhale is an invitation for renewal, and when you align intention with it, you infuse more energy and purpose with each wave of breath.

Yoga is designed to make your body available to as much breath as possible. As you articulate your ujjayi breath and tap into this cycle of expansion and contraction, you unlock the potential within you, and you flood your body with life force energy.

> Take the breath of the new dawn and make it part of you. It will give you strength.
>
> Hopi saying

To perform ujjayi, you'll breathe in and out through nose at the pace of three to four counts on the inhale and three to four counts on the exhale. We use this breath throughout the entire power yoga practice. Whether you are in a sweaty, strengthening sequence or a more restorative practice, the breath will be the same. Here's how to create this breath:

1. Sit down comfortably in easy pose or kneeling.

2. Bring your right index, middle, and ring fingers together and place them at the base of your navel, your belly button.

3. At the bottom of your third finger (ring finger), at your lower abdomen, is the point of engagement for your core lock and where you pull your core in and up. This point is called uddiyana bandha.

4. At the base of your exhales, gently pull your lower abdomen back and lift toward the base of your back ribs. The activation of your lower abdomen is more of an engagement and is not forceful.

5. On your inhales, lift your breath from your low ribs to up and across your collarbones. Feel your breath expand through your entire body.

6. Continue to generate your balanced breath, three to four counts on the inhales and exhales.

7. Bring your left hand in front of your mouth, as if it were a mirror.

8. Breathe in through your nose and feel your ribs flare out in all directions.

9. On your exhale, open your mouth and breathe out as if you were fogging a mirror.

10. Again, inhale through your nostrils and fill up.

11. Open your mouth, exhale, and fog the mirror as you hug your navel back and up.

12. Do this "fogging the mirror" breath three more times.

13. For your fourth round of breath, take a deep inhale through your nose, seal your lips, and exhale as if you are fogging the mirror through your nose. Keep breathing through your nose with your mouth relaxed and closed.

14. Constrict the whisper muscles at the back of your throat to create a sound and texture with each breath. This ocean-like sound becomes a metronome, an audio anchor, to keep you present in your body and with your breath. Just like the engagement of your core lock, the sound and throat constriction of ujjayi breath is subtle and not forceful.

In power yoga, we focus on the power that's available by adding intention, action, and purpose to this automatic function that makes breath mindful. Every breath is an opportunity to create purpose and align with a higher calling of your spirit. With every inhale, you can expand, invite, draw in, and ask. With every exhale, you can

> As breath stills our mind, our energies are free to unhook from the senses and bend inward.
>
> B.K.S. Iyengar

clear out, release, let go, and begin again with a clean slate. It's really that simple when we start to tune in and bring a discipline to the practice. It may not happen right away, but over time, with attention, you start to generate the energy you want to feel.

In your first meditation in chapter 2, you set an intention for your power yoga practice. Recall your one-word intention—your drishti—and let that be your guiding light as you move through the content and practices. Continue to put your attention on what you want to have happen and take your attention off what isn't working as you weave in greater awareness with your breath. Intention and breath work together. As you focus on your higher aim, every breath becomes an opportunity for you to cultivate your power.

Prana

Prana is Sanskrit for "vital life force energy." Yogic philosophy teaches us that prana, or energy, runs through the entire body via thousands of energetic channels (nadis) and is circulated with breath. Yoga poses (asanas) linked with breath (pranayama) clear and cleanse these pathways so that energy and power can flow through the body. This is why you feel good after practicing yoga—you expand the amount of life force energy within you.

Prana and breath work together like a horse and a rider. The breath is like the horse, and it carries the prana, the rider, throughout the body. With conscious deep breaths, you circulate fresh energy throughout your body, which awakens new energy, and clears your body and your mind.   The union of breath and movement helps you build strength, improve flexibility, and find focus. As you expand your breath, you expand your energy. Breath is the pathway for prana and the vehicle for spirit.

TEACHING TIP
Lead With Breath

Power yoga is foremost a breathing practice. If you are not breathing, then you are not doing yoga. Empower your students to ignite breath in a whole new way by cueing each pose, starting with the breath. Call out either the inhale or the exhale, then the name of the pose and the details of the activation and alignment. Guide your students into the next movement using breath.

If you ever feel disconnected or confused, an easy way to realign with your power in the moment is to take a big, deep breath. When you breathe in, you invite new energy, return to your body, and connect back into your purpose. Use the following steps to access this connection:

1. Wherever you are, pause. Feel your feet on the ground. Open your mouth and exhale completely.

2. Seal your lips and take a big inhale through your nose. When your lungs are completely full, hold your breath. Let your breath wash you from the inside as you fill with new energy.

3. After 3 to 5 counts, open your mouth to exhale completely.

A big, deep breath is like giving yourself vital shot of life force energy! Want to take it one step deeper? This time, take these steps.

1. Pause, close your eyes, and ask yourself how you want to feel.

2. When you have your answer, take a big, deep breath and invite in this energy or feeling as you inhale. Use your breath to create the energy you want to feel. A beautiful alchemy happens when we link breath and intention. When we align the breath with a bigger intention, magic happens.

3. On your exhale, let go of anything that's not in alignment with your intention for feeling good. Use this exhale to clear out anything blocking your path to being in your power.

4. Repeat as often as needed. It takes just a few seconds to realign with your breath, and if you choose it, so much more. When you feel disconnected or out of balance, focus on your breath to add intention, purpose, and power.

Foundation

The foundation of your pose is whatever is touching the earth. In standing poses, your feet are the foundation. In inversions, your hands, arms, or head create your foundation. In other poses, your foundation can be your belly, back, or seat. To maximize your power in every yoga pose, first create a strong physical foundation. Once the foundation is stable, you can begin to work the rest of your pose.

Everything in the natural world rises from the ground up. In yoga poses, we mirror the natural elements and build the postures from earth to sky. When you build

> For a tree to become tall, it must grow tough roots among the rocks.
>
> Friedrich Nietzsche

poses from the ground up, stress, imbalance, and rigidity begin to melt away, and you begin to expand in new directions. You don't have to work so hard to control the overall shape because you have firm footing to support you. More structure increases access to power, creativity, and flow. From the earth, you rise and become all that you are designed to be.

Foundation in one simple term is *grounding*. When you are grounded in your body, you can be fully present in this moment. When you establish your foundation physically, you ignite your power. Grounded and present, you are available to align with and realize your bigger intentions physically, emotionally, and spiritually. A solid foundation will take you to new heights. Most power yoga poses are built on the foundation of your feet and hands, so let's get specific to maximize your power in every pose.

Foot and Hand Placement

Proper placement of feet and hands, or whatever is touching the ground, is essential to building a powerful pose. Foot placement determines how your legs relate to the pelvis as well as the impact on your knees, lower back, and so much more. The same goes for poses on the hands—hand placement determines the rotation of shoulders and upper back, which muscles are activated, and which bones are aligned for your energy to flow. If you are not solid and aligned in your base, you pose can feel unbalanced or shaky or lack power. If you ever feel wobbly or frustrated in a pose, try rebuilding your pose from the ground up. All poses start at the foundation.

To establish a solid foundation in standing poses, make sure your feet are parallel, with your big toes facing twelve o'clock, and ground through all four corners of your feet. The four corners of feet are the big toe mound, pinkie toe mound, inner heel, and outer heel (see figure 3.1).

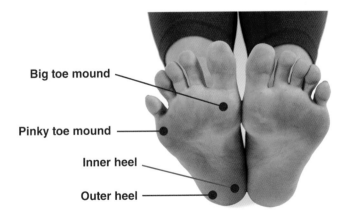

Big toe mound

Pinky toe mound

Inner heel

Outer heel

Figure 3.1 Four corners of the foot.

The alignment of the feet is a general aim because all feet are shaped differently, so experiment to find the alignment that feels most powerful to you. Start at your base and firmly ground through the four corners of the feet. Press down into the earth and lift the arches toward the groin, and your power up into your core. From your core, press back down into the earth through the four corners of your feet. I like to think of it as a plugging into an energetic grid—draw the energy up from the earth and press back down to plug in. This connection creates a stable base for your pose and a platform for growth.

1. Stand at the top of your mat with your feet parallel and aligned at twelve o'clock (see figure 3.2a). You can stand with your feet together or hip-width apart. Hip distance can be measured with your two fists between your feet. A wider base often feels sturdier, especially when you're getting started.

2. Lift your toes off the mat, spread them wide, and press them back into the ground. Take up as much space as you can. Notice how you feel. Notice how you can engage your legs and where you feel most powerful. Notice your connection to your core and the flow of your breath. Note that if the arches of your feet collapse, you'll feel it in your knees. Spread your toes to awaken your feet and access more rooting through the corners.

3. Now experiment with the alignment at your base. Turn your toes out and your heels in so that your knees are facing the outer edges of your mat (see figure 3.2b). Press down through all four corners of your feet and lift your power into your core. Take 5 to 10 deep breaths and notice the impact on your lower back, knees, breath, and drishti. What's different? Do you feel more powerful or less?

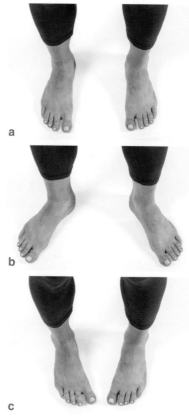

Figure 3.2 Foot placement: *(a)* Neutral position with toes at twelve o'clock, *(b)* toes out and heels in, and *(c)* toes in and heels out.

4. Next, turn your toes in and your heels out so your knees are facing in toward one another and into the center of your mat (see figure 3.2c). Ground down and take 5 to 10 deep breaths. Notice what you feel now. What is the impact on your lower back, knees, breath, and your power?

⑤ Finally, return to your neutral position with your feet parallel. Notice how you feel now.

Where did you feel most powerful? What adjustments can you make to honor your body and create the alignment that best serves you? Use this information to create a powerful base for your standing poses.

Now, try a similar experiment with your hands in downward-facing dog. Discover what feels best for you.

① First, come into downward-facing dog and place your hands at shoulder-width apart or a little wider. Aim your index fingers straight ahead at twelve o'clock (see figure 3.3a). Spread your whole palm on the ground and root down through all your knuckles, especially the index-finger knuckles, as if you were growing deep roots into the earth like a giant oak tree. The knuckles of your index fingers are the main point of pressure of your hands to your mat. If the knuckles start to lift, this is great information coming back from your body that more foundation is available. Now, press down through your hands, activate and firm your arm muscles, and pull your shoulder blades onto your back. Ground down, lift, and take 5 to 10 deep breaths. Notice what you feel. What is the impact on your shoulders, neck, back, and breath?

② Next, turn your index fingers out wide to face the upper corners of your mat (see figure 3.3b). Press down into your hands and activate your arms. Breathe deeply and notice what you feel now. What's the impact on your wrists and elbows? Notice how you can engage your legs and arms, how you can lengthen your spine, and where you feel most powerful. Notice the impact on your breath.

③ Now turn your index fingers into the center of your mat so your elbows are facing to the outer edges of your mat (see figure 3.3c). Ground down and

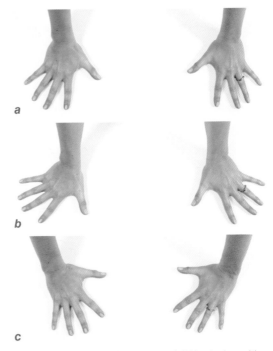

Figure 3.3 Hand placement: *(a)* Neutral position with fingers at twelve o'clock, *(b)* index fingers turned out, and *(c)* index fingers turned in.

take 5 to 10 deep breaths. Notice what you feel now. What is the impact on your wrists, shoulders, and neck? Is your weight distributed equally through your hands and feet or more in one area?

4 Finally, modify your pose to build the structure that works for you. For example, my shoulders are the widest—and tightest—part of my body, so I like to give myself a little more space. I set my hands wider than my shoulders, and I turn my index fingers out slightly. This creates more space and freedom for me in downward-facing dog and through my vinyasa. Experiment to build a solid foundation that creates stability, strength, and flexibility.

Neutral Alignment

Mountain pose (tadasana) is the blueprint for all yoga poses (asanas). It creates neutral alignment within the whole body, and the foundation of tadasana is within every pose. This posture illustrates the strength and sturdiness that is available as you root down into the earth, engage the whole body, and embody the qualities of a mighty mountain. As you ground down into the earth, and lift and expand through your entire body, you align and open physically to allow more power to flow within you.

The alignment and activation of mountain pose helps neutralize stress and imbalance in the body. We all have unique holding patterns—physically and energetically—that show up in the body. These develop over a lifetime, through repetitive motions like spending most of the day on a computer or driving a car, years of the same sport, or holding your child on the same hip. Mountain pose trains the body to be aligned, open, and powerful.

> Keep your eyes on the stars and your feet on the ground.
>
> Theodore Roosevelt

Centerline

The centerline, or the midline, is the union between the right and left sides of the body. It is the structure and energy of the spine and runs from your root all the way to the crown of your head. In yoga philosophy, it's known as the central channel and houses major energy centers. In all poses, you hug into the centerline and extend out from there. Drawing inward pulls your power into your center and creates total body integration and functional stability. You activate and sculpt your muscles by engaging them and hugging them to the bones which enlivens your whole body.

When you move from your center, more mobility becomes possible because you can extend and stretch through the whole body. Hug into your center and expand out with your breath.

Integration

Foundation and integration are created physically through pressing down, lifting up, and pulling in. In every pose, you move from the ground up and from the center out. These actions create a physical union when all parts come together and work together. With your body integrated and ignited, you can start to move with more ease and purpose, and the mind and the body can work as one.

In your power yoga practice, notice your physical patterns or tendencies. You may have a stronger side in some poses or postures where you feel tighter or unsteady. Let every pose be a study of your body and where you can bring things together. Aim for the whole pose, rather than the individual parts. With more integration of your whole body, imbalance will start to melt away, and you will become more coordinated and graceful. There is no end to any pose—work with where you are and express from there.

Foundation and integration are physical, and energetic and spiritual too. Integrity in life is when what you say and what you do are in alignment. When you live from your core values and your intentions, your actions feel natural and harmonious. When you are driven by something at the heart level, other people feel this and your connection to others and the greater good. When selfishness or greed is the fuel for someone's actions, people also feel this—something seems off and generally these pursuits take more effort. With a pure heart and mind, you can take action

---

TEACHING TIP

Speak to the Physical First

When teaching any pose, speak to the physical qualities first. Use clear and simple language to give your students access to the pose in their bodies. Cue breath, foundation, structure, alignment, and activation. When you give students a deeply physical experience, you help create a pathway out of their minds and into their bodies. Guide your students to greater sensation. With embodied experience and muscle memory, they can connect the dots from their experience on the mat to what is possible in their own lives. A physical experience makes the possibilities real, rather than just concepts or yoga philosophy. Your guidance can empower your students to feel the physical benefits and greater possibility in each pose, right now.

that is in alignment with who you are and who you intend to be—in all ways, both on and off the yoga mat.

If you're always struggling to get your footing, you might constantly feel pulled in different directions without a secure foundation. For example, if you're not sure what you want to be doing for work, it's easy to feel stuck or absent in your current job. Motivation and purpose in your work create an outline for you to thrive.

For me, making time on the mat for my physical practice is my foundation for feeling good and centered in my life. I have a history of worrying, spending too much time in my head, and moving quickly, so being grounded in my body is essential for me to be my best. When I don't make time for my practice, it makes a huge difference for how I show up in all other areas my life. I don't feel as settled and purposeful physically, I'm not as focused as I know I can be, and I'm not as mindful in my decision making. I start forgetting things. I notice that I'm more reactive and a little edgy overall—my energy isn't grounded.

I use foundational daily practices for me to clear my head, feel more balanced, and be grounded in my power. My daily practices include sitting in stillness and focusing on my breath, movement, connecting with my partner, and eating foods that serves my energy and health. When I do these things, I'm able to show up in my work for my students and be fully aligned in love with my partner and family. These are all the building blocks that help me thrive. Prioritize what matters and build your strong foundation. Structure your life and yoga practice to empower you to be your best.

> Extend and expand from where you are.
>
> B.K.S. Iyengar

Balanced Action

Sthira Sukha Asanam
Postures should be stable and comfortable.
The Yoga Sutras of Patanjali: Yoga Sutra 2.46

This thread of wisdom from *The Yoga Sutras of Patanjali* reveals that the aim of each yoga pose is to create balanced action or cultivate a balance of strength and ease. *Sthira* translates to "steady, hard, or strong." *Sukha* means "soft, sweetness, or ease." *Asanam* means "wholeness, the seat or pose of the yogi, or the whole community of the body."

In yoga, you can't just power through your practice. When you strengthen one part of your body, you allow another part to release. Both strength and surrender are required. In every pose, we activate certain muscles and allow others to relax.

What you eat matters and becomes the fuel for your yoga practice and your life. Eating healthy, nutrient-dense foods serves as a platform for feeling good and loving your body.

Leafy greens are power foods. Aim to include something green in every meal to cleanse your body and create the foundation for your vibrant health. What you eat becomes the cells in your body and the energy you use to live your life.

Like straight shots of vitality, most green vegetables contain more than 18 vitamins and minerals that promote stronger bones, provide a healthy dose of plant-based protein, and deliver vital energy straight from the earth to your body and your cells. The simple shift of adding more greens into the diet creates a powerful, transformative effect on your entire body. Build your foundation with life-giving foods. Use the following tips:

- Throw in a handful of spinach with your eggs in the morning.
- Add a side of veggies instead of fries while out to lunch.
- Have a salad of raw greens and vegetables before your dinner.
- Have a big, green salad for lunch.
- Drink a green juice or green smoothie as midafternoon snack.
- Sub a side of spinach in place of potatoes or bread at dinner.

You create power by using your entire body, all the parts that make you whole, and invite everything into one holistic and balanced practice.

For example, in tadasana, if you are not stable in your feet or your muscles are not engaged and drawing into your center, your whole pose can feel wobbly. With too much ease or softness, strength and form are missing. However, if you are too rigid or forceful in a pose, you can hurt yourself, and your movements can be choppy or reactive. Too much tightness or rigidity won't allow for breath or flow of energy or for your body to mold in a new way. When one energy is dominant either in your body or your life, you can bring the opposite in your power yoga practice to cultivate balance.

In yoga poses, you can balance both drive and effort while honoring your sensitivity. Each yoga pose is a chance to build power and learn when to let go, how to respect your body's limitations, and how to stay comfortable in the discomfort of growth. This ongoing communication is unique to each person, in each practice and every breath. We all experience different factors that contribute to our flexibility, clarity, and power daily. In your power yoga practice, you can play the edge between extremes and literally find the balance that works for you. It's not how far you go in the pose but who you are and the energy you create within the pose that matters.

We are always searching for balance—in our work, relationships, and bodies. By practicing balanced action within each yoga pose, you can better understand how to create the same results in other areas of your life. For example, off the mat, too much sukha can show up as always running late, being flighty or forgetful, or feeling a lack of direction or purpose. If the energy of sukha is dominant in your life, try adding in structure that cultivates stability and grounded energy. This could look like scheduling your daily yoga practice in your calendar or holding yourself accountable to building strength in your 28-day power yoga plan.

> **Life is a balance of holding on and letting go.**
>
> Rumi

An abundance of sthira can look like needing things to always go according to plan, being hyper-detailed, obsessing about your workouts or diet, or being fixed in your positions, and fiercely defending your point of view. This energy of rigidity and rightness takes a toll physically, showing up as stress, tension, and the inability to chill out. Adding in a practice of surrender and release, like the cool-down sequences in this book or a regular meditation practice, can open you to more joy, freedom, and ease.

Grounded in the Moment

Foundation looks different in each moment, depending on the circumstances you are working with, what yoga pose you are in, or where you are in your practice both on and off the mat. Creating your foundation is a moment-to-moment dance.

Two questions that can help you establish your foundation and your next step for more power are:

What is actually happening?

What structure will empower you right now?

Remember, right now is when yoga happens, and it's the only time we have access to power. When you can get to what is real, what's happening underneath the movement or emotion, you can get to the clear next steps that will empower you moving forward. Seek to understand what is real and get to the facts.

Let's take a deeper look at these questions and how they could show up on the mat. Standing balancing poses are great opportunities to practice building a strong foundation. Let's use dancer pose (natarajasana) and two common ways of reestablishing your base.

If you are standing on your left foot and keep falling over to the left, your body and this pattern are giving you a lot of feedback about what's happening at your foundation. To create stability, root down more through your left big toe mound, anchor down through your standing foot, and hug your outer (left) shin into your centerline.

Grab your journal and a pen and reflect on these questions about your foundation in your yoga practice and your life.

- When do you feel most grounded? Where? Whom are you with?
- In what yoga poses do you feel most stable?
- What poses make you feel off balance?
- What contributes to you feeling centered? What do you need to feel grounded and in your power?
- How do you practice coming back to your center and reclaiming your power in the present moment?
- Where can you cultivate greater connection to others in your life?
- What daily practices, rituals or habits create the foundation for you being your best?

In the same pose, still balanced on your left foot, the opposite can happen. If you keep falling to the right, you could be splaying your lifted right leg out too far to the right and pulling yourself off center. What's missing is drawing your energy to your centerline as you kick your lifted leg back.

As you look for what is happening at your foundation, you will get specific and direct feedback coming from the body. Ask these two questions: What's actually happening? What structure will empower you right now? This is a quick way to align with what's most important in the moment and get grounded in your power. The answers are often physical but can sometimes be energetic or emotional.

For example, during my first five years of practicing power yoga, every time my teacher called eagle pose, I would think, "Oh my God. I hate this pose. I don't want to do this pose. I feel so tight in this pose." As a result, it would be a tough experience for me—10 breaths felt like an eternity.

> **Make the best use of what's in your power and take the rest as it happens.**
>
> Epictetus

Before I even went into the pose, fear, anxiety, and anger were taking over. I was taking up all the space with my own energy—the resistance took over before I got into the physical shape. Sthira was dominating, and I wasn't allowing for the sukha, the ease to come with the pose or my experience to unfold naturally.

The structure that I needed for my eagle pose was being in a clear space. I needed to clear out the clutter of my body and mind to be able to access the benefits of the pose. Once I started adapting my pose to be easier on my body and became more balanced in my approach, I found great benefit in the pose that I resisted for so long. It took me five years to realize that *I* was the block in letting my eagle pose happen.

The same questions, the same reflection, led me to this insight. I had to listen to what was happening in my body and adjust who I was being in my practice and my approach in order to access the results. We have so much direct feedback coming back from the body in yoga poses. When we lean in and listen, we can take our experience on the mat and expand this knowledge and learning into life.

Energy Locks

Bandhas are subtle energetic locks within the body that help with longer holds, navigating newer poses, transitions, and floating. In Sanskrit, *bandha* means "to lock, to hold, or to tighten." The three main locks used in power yoga are located along the centerline, and a fourth lock ties them all together. Engaging your bandhas is a practice of managing internal energy and power and helps generate concentration, clarity, and steadiness within each pose. The three main locks are shown in figure 3.4.

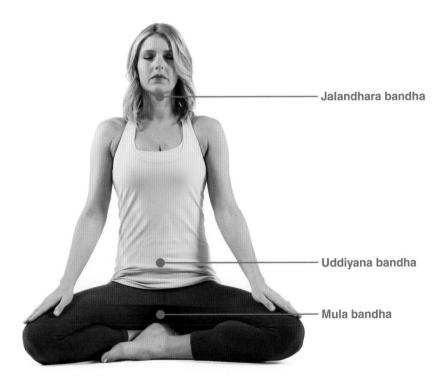

Jalandhara bandha

Uddiyana bandha

Mula bandha

Figure. 3.4 Bandhas: mula bandha or root lock, uddiyana bandha or core lock, and jalandhara bandha or chin lock.

❶ *Mula bandha*: This lock is located at the base of the spine. For women, activating the root lock is similar to doing a Kegel, and for men it's described as comparable to cutting off the flow of urine. Engaging this lock gives you access to lightness through transitions and inversions.

❷ *Uddiyana bandha*: This lock is located at the lower abdomen. To engage your core lock, gently pull your lower abdomen in and up. This lock builds core strength, stabilizes the spine, tones the abs, and protects the lower back.

❸ *Jalandhara bandha*: This lock is located at the throat. To activate your chin lock, lift your chest and drop your chin down, like you are creating a double chin. This lock helps contain your energy in your lower body and activates the energy center within your throat and the muscles of your neck.

The main bandha we use in power yoga is the core lock, uddiyana bandha, and we activate it in every pose. It's a gentle, rhythmic engagement and is not forceful. This energetic lock unites the upper and lower halves of the body and helps creates total body integration as well a sense of lightness.

EXERCISE: CORE LOCK

To activate core lock, bring your right index, middle, and ring fingers together and place them at the base of your navel. At the bottom of your third finger is the point of activation for your core lock. At the base of your exhales, gently pull your lower abdomen toward your spine and lift to the middle of your back, behind your heart. It's a steady engagement, not a fierce drawing back.

As you activate your core lock and lift your lower abdomen up and in, your breath can lift and expand into your chest and upper torso. Notice if your breath starts to wane at any time in your practice, and use your core lock to help bring back your powerful ujjayi breath. At the base of your exhales, aim to fully engage your core lock. On your inhales, keep the gentle engagement at about 20 percent. This is not a perfect science; it's a more general aim and rhythmic reminder of your power. Ignite your core and empower your deep, full breath.

Bandhas are energetic, and it may take a while to build this awareness and connection within your practice. If you are newer to yoga or haven't been physical in a while, start with focusing on your hands and feet and building a strong foundation in every pose. For example, in downward-facing dog, firmly press your hands into your mat and pull your shoulders back. The pressing and pulling will help to develop integration and core awareness. If you are a more seasoned practitioner, try building awareness and activation of your bandhas. Learning is available at every level.

A lot of people come to yoga seeking relief from back pain. If you're not integrated at the core, you move from individual parts of your body and the exterior which create a disintegration within the body. Not moving from your center can lead to back pain or other injuries. Uddiyana bandha is foundational for building strength and moving with power from your center.

Chakras

The seven chakras, or energy centers, exist along the spine or the centerline of the body. They run from the root to the top of the head. *Chakra* means "wheel" or "vortex" of energy. Each chakra has its own vibrational frequency and affects our physical, mental, emotional, and spiritual well-being.

The chakras are extremely receptive to what we think, feel, and repeatedly do. When energy is blocked, either through overactivity or atrophy, it can show up physically and emotionally. The chakras cannot be seen or touched; they are experienced and felt. They affect our perceptions, personality, feelings, and choices.

Each chakra governs certain aspects of our lives and is tied to specific areas of the body as well as to emotions, natural elements, and colors. We can use this ancient map of our energy centers to inform our yoga practices and daily rituals to cultivate more healing, purpose, and inner peace. Table 3.1 provides an overview of each chakra, the qualities, and various practices to help balance your subtle energy. Notice what descriptions ring true for you and how you can use this information to adapt your yoga practice to honor your needs, work with specific areas of the body as you unlock power within the chakras.

> The chakras are very intelligent— they are like the software of the whole computer body.
>
> Dharma Mittra

Table 3.1 The Chakras: A Map of the Major Energy Centers

Chakra	Location	Color	Element	Governs	
Crown chakra: understanding, spirituality, sahasrara	Top of the head, crown, pineal gland	White	The Cosmos	Belief systems, faith, higher power, divinity, self-knowledge, open-mindedness, ability to question, connection to spirit	
Third- eye chakra: sight, intuition,ajna	Forehead, brow, third eye, face, sinus cavity, pituitary gland	Purple or indigo	Light	Intuition, imagination, wisdom, knowledge, insight, instinct, dreams, vision, memory	
Throat chakra: communication visshudha	Throat, neck, jaw, thyroid	Bright blue	Sound	Self-expression, voice, language, listening, communication	
Heart chakra: love anahata	Heart, chest, cardiac plexus, arms, shoulders, thymus gland	Green	Air	Love, relationships, compassion, empathy, romance, friendship, self-love, giving and receiving, immunity, devotion	
Solar plexus (or core) chakra: transformation manipura	Solar plexus, torso, abdomen, pancreas	Yellow	Fire	Personal power, life purpose, career, individuality, passion, motivation	
Sacral chakra: connection svadhisthana	Lower abdomen, sacral plexus, hips, pelvis, and ovaries or testes	Orange	Water	Pleasure, well-being, sexuality, play, creativity, desire, movement, emotion	
Root chakra: foundation muladhara	Base of spine, feet, legs, toes, heels, ankles, knees, thighs, calves, adrenals	Red	Earth	Home, health, family safety, support, finances, appropriate boundaries	

Emotional issues	Poses for power	Practices	Affirmations
Vanity, over-intellectualization, spiritual addiction, confusion, rigid belief systems, skepticism, apathy	Poses and practice that help you to integrate your entire body and being, and connect to your inner truth: meditation, anjali mudra, savasana	Meditation, mantra, gratitude, and spiritual discipline	I am open to new ideas. I trust the process. The world is my teacher. I acknowledge the presence of spirit in my life. I release fear and doubt and I accept that my life is blessed.
Poor memory, lack of imagination or ability to think outside the box, denial, attention deficit, concentration, excessive daydreaming, lack of follow-through	Poses that help you set your vision and build awareness: sukhasana, child's pose, eagle, airplane, dolphin, forearm balance	Meditation, drishti, pranayama, and spending time in nature	I see clearly. I am open to the wisdom within. I can manifest my vision. I use my intuition and intelligence to light my way forward.
Expressing feelings and truth, ability to speak up, timing and rhythm, discernment, shame, repressed emotions	Postures that open your throat and neck and empower you to communicate clearly and honestly: neck rolls, shoulder stand, fish pose, legs-up-the-wall	Singing, chanting, head and neck alignment, pranayama, and inquiry	I hear and speak the truth. I share my feelings with ease. I listen to my inner guidance. My voice is necessary.
Inner peace, joy, love, acceptance, loneliness, jealousy, judgement, isolation, sadness	Poses and sequences that get your heart pumping, improve your cardiovascular health, open your shoulders and chest: lunge with a bind, flip dog, upward dog, bow, bridge, wheel	Breath, pranayama, self-care and self-reflection	I am love. I am worthy of love. I am loving to myself and others. There is an infinite supply of love.
Inner strength, self-worth, confidence, doubt, hyperactivity or laziness, stubbornness, responsibility	Poses that require you to take a risk and build confidence, and poses that stimulate core energy and abdominal strength: boat pose, plank pose, chair twist, handstand, crow pose, wheel	Fire ceremony to burn what you no longer need and self-inquiry	I can do it. I honor the power within me. I am whole. I am worthy of a good life.
Emotional intelligence, ability to experience pleasure, setting boundaries, balance of work and play, ability to accept change, gratitude, follow-through	Hip-opening poses that help you loosen tightness and get your energy flowing: low lunge, goddess, wide-leg forward fold, reclined bound angle, frog	Swimming, being in water, artwork, and play	I deserve pleasure and joy. I embrace and celebrate my sexuality. I move easily and effortlessly. I allow abundance and goodness into my life.
Survival, self-worth, confidence, self-esteem, financial independence, anger, aggression, defensiveness, belonging	Grounded and stable standing poses that help activate and empower your foundation and whole body: warrior I, II, reverse warrior, extended side angle, yogi squat, tree pose	Gardening, inquiry, eating grounding foods, and massage and bodywork	I am safe. I love my body. I am supported. All my needs are being met. I choose life. I accept myself as I am.

Heat

Heat in the power yoga practice is strengthening, cleansing, and purifying. Heat is the key element that sets power yoga apart from other styles of yoga. On the mat, we'll focus on heat-building poses and sequences, like sun salutations, standing poses, and twists that will stoke your inner fire and make you feel alive. Heat softens the tissues and muscles and makes the body more malleable. When glass is cold, you can't reshape it, but if you apply heat to glass, you can bend and meld it into something new and beautiful. You have to bring heat to glass to access this magic. It's the same with the body. When you heat the body, you can shape it in ways that might not seem possible when you first start your yoga practice. Heat melts away layers of resistance and old holding patterns, physically and energetically. We create heat physically in power yoga in three main ways.

❶ Heat-building breath (ujjayi pranayama)

❷ Linking breath with movement (vinyasa)

❸ Heating the yoga room to between 85 and 95 degrees

By building inner heat through breath and movement, you get deeper into your body and open communication and understanding from within that doesn't happen on the surface. When you practice in a heated room, heat becomes a tool to get into the body faster, making an effective and efficient practice. Heat softens the tissues and muscles and makes the body more receptive. You start to melt away old patterns, tightness, and limiting perceptions of your body as you develop new strength, endurance, confidence, and move in ways you once thought couldn't happen.

> The cure for anything is saltwater: sweat, tears, or the sea.
>
> Isak Dinesen

Sweat naturally heals the body by releasing toxins. When you start to sweat, your muscles get pliable, helping you feel the results of your practice faster. We live in such a fast-paced and toxic environment today that it's important to be in some sort of practice of detoxing and purifying on a regular basis. A heated yoga room can be uncomfortable at first, but once you access that power of purification, it feels good. The body is always seeking homeostasis, so as you get into your ritual of practicing in the cleansing heat, you'll find that your body will be pulled toward this practice of sweating and coming back to your natural state.

Heat is life-giving, creating regeneration and rebirth. The heat of the sun gives life to all the earth, and plants always bend toward the light. The fire element in yoga practice helps burn off old habits, limiting beliefs, fear, resistance, extra weight, old relationships, what's not serving you, and impurities or excess that gets picked up from living life.

Tapas is one of the five niyamas outlined in the *Yoga Sutras of Pantajali*, and can defined as "fiery discipline" or "zeal." It teaches us that power builds through repetition. As you cultivate your inner fire, your spiritual energy grows. Tremendous energy is unlocked in yoga practice through being consistent and disciplined. As you come to your mat each day, you start to build strength and start to believe in your potential. When you feel good in your body, your confidence will soar both on and off the mat, and stress and discomfort will start to melt away, igniting your personal power.

Building discipline into your daily routine creates a path to accomplishing your goals, increases personal accountability, and gets the mind, body, and heart working as one. This can be simple, like carving out time each morning for yoga practice or meditation or choosing to eat healthy, energy-boosting foods. As you commit to new practices that serve you, energy builds, and you start to see the results. When you say yes to a new way now, you start to release old habits or ways of being that are outdated and no longer needed. You'll feel yourself start to bend toward the light as you begin to burn brighter.

Tapas is a tool for transformation and should be approached with passion and commitment, rather than obligation, guilt, or restriction. You want the heat to be steady and life affirming, so it's important to maintain a sense of balance with the other elements, breath, overall energy, and alignment with your intentions. Too much fire, or too much too fast, can cause burnout.

> Yoga is for internal cleansing, not external exercising. Yoga means true self-knowledge.
>
> Sri K. Pattabhi Jois

Practicing heat-boosting power yoga not only helps you go deeper and heal but also pushes you out of your comfort zone. It's easy to build a very comfortable life and avoid situations that don't feel good. Staying in a safe place in any area of life for too long creates stuck energy and disconnects you from life force energy for the body, mind, and spirit. You can access a new level of expression and growth when you start to feel stretched, pulled, or like the heat is being turned up. Our spirits grow when we extend beyond our perceived limitations and into new space. Heat can help you disrupt the way things have been, discover your edge, and move into what can be now. However, once you are out of your comfort zone, it's important to be able to stay in that state for a while instead of retreating to what you know, to what is easy. Big things happen when you can challenge yourself to be uncomfortable, and it's essential for growth. For example, the challenge of balancing on one foot in a heated room, with sweat running down your face, forces you to focus on your drishti to breathe through the discomfort of the moment.

Tapas teaches you how to stay while you're uncomfortable. This is such an incredible tool to have in a modern, busy life—not to run when the heat kicks in. When we feel physical discomfort and stay in the challenge, we build energetic and muscular memory that being uncomfortable is OK. It's an important part of rewiring your body and seeing things in a new way. When you can be with things as they are and don't have to fix, micromanage, or change them, you free your energy. By staying in the fire, and letting things be as they are, whether it's a heated room for 60 minutes; a deep, long hip-opening pose; or a challenging conversation with a

> In the middle of difficulty lies opportunity.
>
> Albert Einstein

TEACHING TIP

Stoke the Fire

As teacher, be willing to push your students beyond their comfort zones. To build new energy, you have to extend past your normal limits. This stress is key to growth. Look for the winnable gaps between where your students are now and what you know is possible for them and move your students to their edges. Don't be afraid to hold your students in the fire, where their whole bodies are radiating heat. Every yoga pose is an opportunity for your students to explore their limits, build power, and learn how to stay comfortable in the discomfort of growth. Guide your students with both certainty and compassion so they can explore how to respond powerfully when things get uncomfortable and how to return to center without coming undone.

Take out your journal and something to write with and answer these open-ended questions about where you can access the power of heat in your practice and your life.

Where do you feel the heat being turned up in your life?

Where do you feel most depleted in your life right now?

What are you ready to say good-bye to in your life because it no longer serves you?

What fuels and inspires you?

What are you committed to now?

What are you ready for?

loved one, you begin to tap into a deep reservoir of inner power. This will serve you at work, in your relationships, and in a sweaty power yoga practice.

I've developed this skill on the mat and use it to stay centered when the heat gets turned up in my life. When I move through tough conversations or life transitions or when I'm feeling stretched out in all directions with overcommitment, the clarity I cultivated in power yoga helps me stay grounded in patience and love. When I give into anger or am overwhelmed, I lose my power. I know that if I stay patient in the middle of the fire, there are rewards waiting on the other side.

Sometimes life calls for total disruption or destruction. Tapas reminds us that everything changes and nothing in life is permanent. These times of major challenge and trial are ripe for rebirth and transformation. The moments you choose to stay in the discomfort and meet your challenges head-on can be some of the most defining and liberating moments directing you to your true path. Yoga teaches us to trust the process—trust discomfort, the stumbles, and the lows—and use these experiences to align with the light. We learn through contrast and experience; you have to know the darkness to know the light. When you've endured great challenge in life, you know that you can persevere, withstand, and eventually thrive. There is no need to run and hide when the heat gets turned up. Feel what you feel and choose to stay in the fire and see what emerges on the other side.

> To be fully alive, fully human, and completely awake is to be continually thrown out of the nest.
>
> Pema Chodron

Tapas teaches us the power in staying—staying in the pose, staying with your breath, and staying with your consistent practice. Activate the healing power of tapas within your practice, step into the cleansing heat, and let the fire transform you.

Flow

In power yoga, we coordinate yoga poses with breath. The marriage of breath and movement starts to smooth away any excess energy in the body and creates a mindfulness in motion. *Vinyasa* in Sanskrit means "flow." This is where physical and mental stress and tension begin to melt away as your body and breath take the lead. Fluid and balanced movements create a soothing, calm energy and can reduce anxiety, depression, and fear while building focus and concentration.

When you surrender mental energy to your breath and physical process, your practice becomes a meditation in motion. When you are fully committed to the physical experience, synchronizing movement with breath at a steady pace, you begin to flow seamlessly from one pose to the next. You start to smooth out resistance in the body and the mind.

Because the breath carries prana throughout your entire body, linking breath with movement amplifies the life-affirming results. However, if your movements don't match the breath or you override breath by forcing, you can create blocks, agitation, or tension within the body. You are working against your nature, your breath. The magic happens in the cocreation of body and breath.

Flow is the embodiment of the water quality. Water is one of the most powerful forces on earth, dancing around or through any obstacles in its path. It smooths over resistance, like rocks and branches, through its gentle yet persistent power. It's always moving forward

> The rhythm of the body, the melody of the mind, and the harmony of the soul create the symphony of life.
>
> B.K.S. Iyengar

and is at times destructive if necessary while it lets nothing disrupt its purposeful flow. Water brings the right amount of effort and is the balance of strength and softness. Like water, flow is the embodiment of ease and the absence of resistance.

Flow gives us an opportunity to refresh and reset. When we are on the mat, away from our stressful lives, we can start to dive into a deeper, more healing element within ourselves and wash away some of the tension and tightness that comes from living life today.

Flow is possible when you are clear in your vision (your drishti), aligned with your breath, and open and receptive to life as it happening. Yoga helps us to tune in to the body and become more aware when tension and resistance arise within us. These sensations are cues that signal more ease is available through letting go. When we become fixed in our positions, attached to the way we think things need to be, or try to make something happen before it's time, we lose the ability to flow. When we hold on too tight, brace, or try to force an outcome, we cut off the flow of life force energy—physically, mentally, emotionally, and spiritually. You become the block in the stream rather than the river.

> Life is a series of natural and spontaneous changes. Don't resist them; that only creates sorrow. Let reality be reality. Let things flow naturally forward in whatever way they like.
>
> Lao Tzu

THE IMPORTANCE OF STAYING HYDRATED

Our bodies are mostly water, which is why hydration is essential for proper organ function, smooth digestion, and overall optimal health and energy. When you're hydrated, your muscles and joints are lubricated, and you can go longer without "hitting a wall" in your power yoga practice.

Water helps move everything through your system and flushes out toxins. When the body is cleansing regularly, more vital energy is available to live life fully in your power. Water helps transport oxygen and other essential nutrients to your cells and improves blood flow. It plumps up skin cells, making your skin more clear, clean, and luminous!

A good rule of thumb is to drink eight glasses of water per day or more, depending on how much activity and yoga you're doing. If you sweat a lot in your power yoga practice, remember to add electrolytes like lemon. Note: If you're feeling thirsty, then you are already dehydrated.

Take out a piece of paper or your journal and something to write with and answer these open-ended questions about how you can access more flow.

What changes are you resisting?

Are you trying to control outcomes in your life? If yes, where?

Where do you feel stuck? In your yoga practice? In your work? In your relationships?

Where can you bring ease and flow into your life?

Where or when do you feel most energized and alive?

Where can you let go more?

When you feel you need to control a situation or feel yourself trying too hard, whether in a conversation or in a yoga pose, this is a cue that another way is possible and to look for a path of less resistance. Less effort means more energy for you to use in a way that serves you, your life, and your bigger intentions.

It's a moment-to-moment practice to return to your flow and move from your center. It comes from letting go of the way things need to be and accepting things the way they are. Letting go allows your life to flow.

Being in the flow is similar to the experience of an elite athlete in the zone—when all the forces come together, and they become one with the elements. Because power yoga is such a deeply physical practice, we can tap into a similar zone (flow) every time we step on mat. As we surrender mentally, the union of breath and body takes the power yoga practice from something you do into something that you are.

The on-the-mat experience gives us an embodied understanding of what it feels like to live in alignment with ease, purpose, and inner strength. You are tuned in and can recognize when elements are not aligned—when resistance or blocks emerge—and when to course-correct to maximize your energy and results. Your power yoga practice is an opportunity to hone in and focus on the results you want to create—in all areas of your life—every time you step onto your yoga mat. Finding

TEACHING TIP
Stay One Beat Ahead

Stay one beat ahead of your students' practice with your cues. Guide your students into the next movement so that they can have the physical experience of ease, flow, and power. If they are waiting for your cues, you can create a choppy and disjointed experience physically, energetically, and emotionally. Let your words open the pathway for them to flow.

your flow ties your practice and life together, taking both into another realm. You start to tap into your artistry, your zone, and the realization of the life that you want to live. Being in your flow comes from living in alignment with what makes you feel most alive.

For me, being in my flow means being graceful and purposeful in everything that I do. Anxiety, anger, and being overwhelmed are the opposite of how I want to feel, so when those energies inevitably creep into my life, it's my cue from my body to slow things down, realign, and get back to my center, where I can be in my zone. In this space, I choose to respond rather than react. In my flow, I know I am more kind to myself and to others, I pay attention, I'm more loving with my family, and I'm able to show up fully in my work as I share yoga with my students on and off the mat.

Being in your flow is living in alignment with your higher vision, being fully present and in your power. It's not something you do once. A moment-to-moment practice creates a powerful way of living. Embodying the water quality empowers you to be more available to be in dance of life.

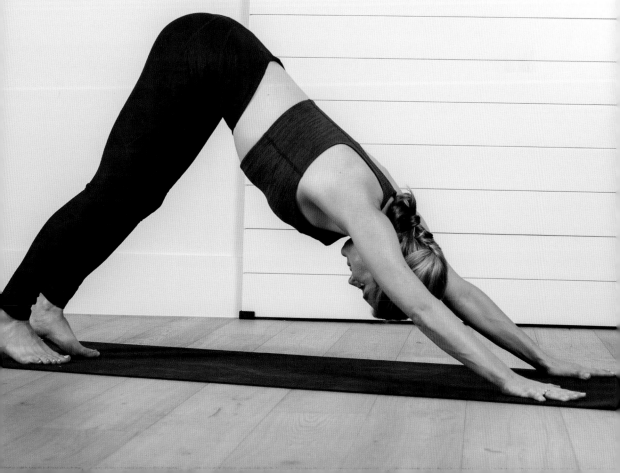

CHAPTER 4

Warm-Up Poses and Sequences

I have been a seeker, and I still am, but I stopped asking the books and the stars. I started listening to the teaching of my soul.

Rumi

In this chapter, we'll look at the building blocks for your power yoga practice. I'll also share how to start each power yoga practice with opening poses, sequences, and sun salutations.

How you begin sets the tone for your experience. The first pose helps you lay the groundwork, awaken your breath, and shift your awareness inward. The opening sequence and sun salutations will help you clear your mind and light your inner fire. As you tune in to your body and breath, you'll bring all your energy into the present moment. You can let go of the rest of your day and anything that has been weighing you down or pulling at your power. Shift your attention to what's right here and now and begin your transformative journey.

Opening Poses

The first pose on your mat is your opportunity to tune into your body and tune out the rest of your day. You can go within and integrate your body, mind, and spirit as your energy settles. The first pose also lays the foundation for the coming sequence. These poses are gentle, comfortable, and allow you to connect you with your breath. Opening poses can be held anywhere from one to five minutes. It may take some time to create this connection from your head to your full body, so allow yourself the space and time to fully embody your breath before you move on. Once you feel and understand the rhythm of your breath, then you start to add movement. You can return to your opening pose throughout your practice to rest, recenter, or reignite your breath.

Child's Pose
Balasana

About the Pose

This pose awakens the connection between the breath and body and sends calming energy through all the muscles. It's an opportunity to get grounded, go inward, and to come out of your busy mind and into your body by awakening your breath.

Child's pose is always available during your practice. If your breath becomes labored from too much effort, or lazy from distraction, use child's pose to reconnect to your breath and your intention for your practice. You can also use it to simply rest. This pose gives you an opportunity to surrender and center.

Alignment

- At the back of your mat, bring your big toes together. Widen your knees to the edges of your mat, wide enough so that your ribs can settle between your thighs.
- Press your hips back to rest on your heels. Extend your arms forward, spread your fingers, and anchor your knuckles into the mat.
- Rest your forehead on the mat and allow your shoulders to soften.
- Fill the space between your ribs with each inhale. As you complete your exhale, gently lift your lower abdomen in and up.

Modifications and Adaptations

Tented fingers: Stay with your breath and bring your attention to your hands. Press down through your fingertips and lift through the center of your palms. Activate your arm muscles by squeezing from skin to muscle to bone and lift your armpits toward the sky.

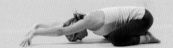

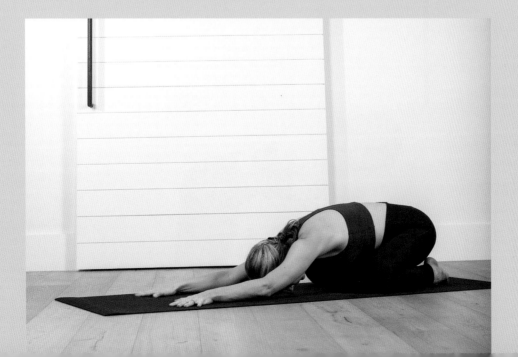

Tabletop

About the Pose

Tabletop is a neutral pose done on all fours. It can be used as a modification for downward-facing dog, a resting pose, or as a transition.

Alignment

- Come to your hands and knees, stack your shoulders over your wrists and your hips over your knees. Either press the tops of your feet into the mat or tuck your toes under for more support.

- On all fours, extend your tailbone to the back of your mat as you lengthen your crown forward.

- Pull the base of your palms toward your knees and your knees toward your palms to ignite your core and lift your low belly.

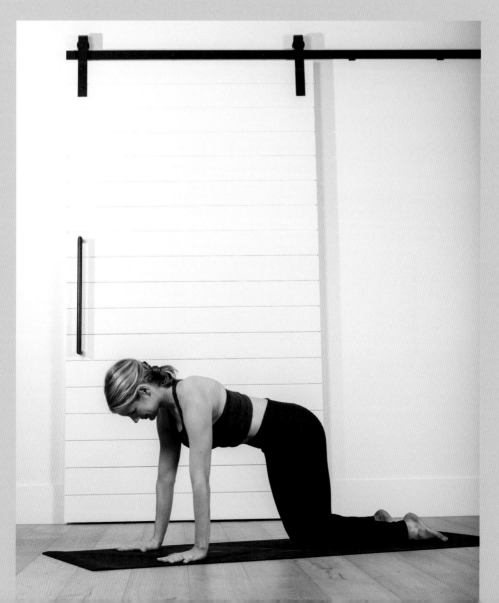

Modifications and Adaptations

These modifications add core strength, balance, glute strength, and heat to the tabletop foundation.

- *Extended tabletop*: Tuck your toes to create more stability and hug your outer shins in. Lift and engage your core. Reach your right arm forward at shoulder height, with your thumb up, and open your fingers. Extend your left heel to the back wall at hip level and flex your foot. Hold for 5 to 10 breaths or add more strength-building elements. Repeat on the other side.

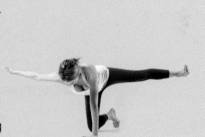

- *Awkward airplane*: Reengage through your lower abdomen and extend your right arm toward the wall on the right. Extend straight out from your shoulder with your palm facing the floor. Firm your left leg and kick your heel to the left at hip level, your toes facing the front of your mat. Lift from your butt and your back body. Hold for 5 to 10 deep breaths. Return to tabletop and switch sides.

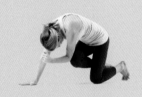

- *Tabletop crunches*: This variation of tabletop incorporates the actions of cat and cow, emphasizes breath, and builds core strength and balance. Come to tabletop on your hands and knees. Lift your lower abdomen up and in so your core is engaged and your back is long. Inhale into extended tabletop. On your exhale, touch your right elbow to your left knee. Round your back in a cat pose, and lift your core. With your inhale, extend your right arm forward and your left leg back. Exhale and hug into the crunch. Keep going one breath per movement for 5 rounds or more. Return to all fours. Repeat on the other side (shown).

Cat and Cow
Marjaryasana/Bitilasana

About the Pose
Cat and cow are two different poses usually done together, linked with breath. This sequence gently opens and awakens the energy along the spine as you link breath with movement. It increases flexibility of the whole spine, neck and shoulders.

Alignment
- Come to tabletop on your hands and knees, with your hands rooted under your shoulders and your knees under your hips. Tuck your toes to help you stabilize and hug your lower belly up and in.
- With your inhale, relax your belly down, draw your shoulder blades together to open across your chest, and lift your gaze as you go into cow pose.

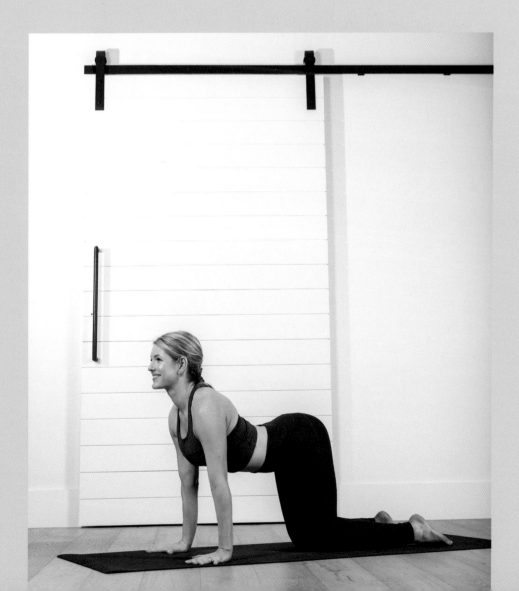

- With your exhale, arch your back and round into cat pose. Press the ground away and tuck your chin to your chest.

- Inhale to cow pose and exhale to cat pose. Keep going one breath per movement for 10 rounds or more. Return to tabletop.

Modifications and Adaptations

As you move with breath, notice what your body calls for. Feel free to add any movements, like moving your hips side-to-side, that feel good to you and honor your unique needs.

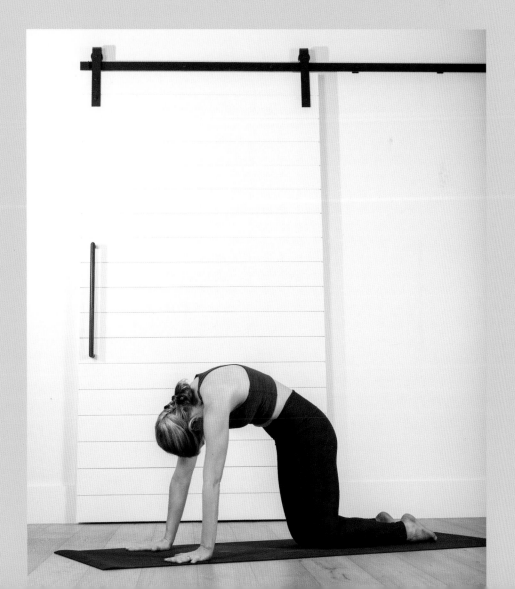

Reclined Bound Angle

Supta Baddha Konasana

About the Pose

This classic restorative and neutralizing pose, also called reclined butterfly, soothes the nervous system because it allows the body to rest on the earth. It opens and stimulates the abdominal organs and heart and stretches the inner thighs and groin. Let your whole body be supported by the earth beneath you as you start your practice or use this as a resting pose during class or toward the end of your practice.

Alignment

- Lie on your back, bring the soles of your feet together, and spread your knees wide.
- Lengthen your tailbone toward your heels to elongate and relax your lower back.
- Extend your arms out to your sides with your palms facing up or bring one hand to your heart and one hand to your low belly.
- Close your eyes and tune in to your breath.

Modifications and Adaptations

If you feel strain on your knees or lower back, you can move your feet further away from your groin or place blocks under your knees for support. If an area of your body calls out for a little more love as you begin, feel free to place both hands there as you generate your breath.

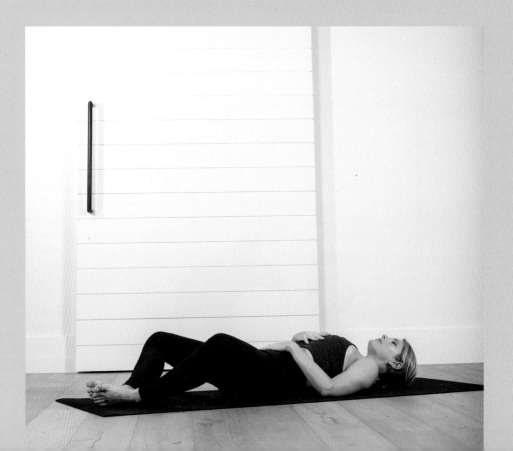

Supine Twist

Jathara Parivartanasana

About the Pose

This gentle twist unwinds and strengthens the middle and lower back and core. It rinses the organs of the midsection, boosting overall health and well-being. It's a great opening or closing pose.

Alignment

- Lie down and gently pull your right knee to your chest as you extend your left leg long. Hug your right knee toward your armpit and flex all your toes.
- Hold your right knee with your left hand, and twist it across to the left side of your mat.
- Extend your right arm long and gaze over your right shoulder.
- With your inhales, lengthen through the side of your body.
- With your exhales, pull your navel back toward your spine and twist from your center.
- Unwind, come through the center, and repeat on the other side (shown).

Modifications and Adaptations

Twist with eagle legs: On your back, wrap your right leg over your left thigh and create eagle legs. Twist both legs to the left, turn your gaze over your right shoulder, and extend your right arm straight out from your shoulder. Place your left hand to the top of your right leg to help deepen your twist. Repeat on the left side (shown).

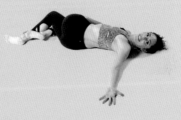

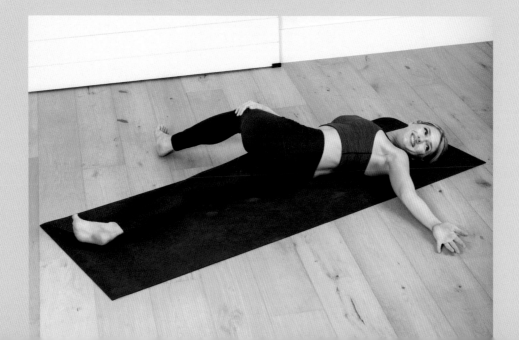

Easy Pose
Sukhasana

Sukhasana is a great way to start your practice and bridge your thinking mind to your feeling body. It is the main pose for seated meditation. This pose calms the brain, lengthens and strengthens the back muscles and spine, opens the hips, and stretches the knees and ankles. Easy pose creates a sense of grounding as you root down through your sitting bones and lift your chest toward the sky, and encourages healthy overall posture. In many cultures, sitting on the floor is common, but in the West, this seated pose can feel challenging.

Alignment

- Sit on the floor, a block, or on a blanket so that your hips are higher than your knees.
- Cross your shins, widen your knees apart, and slide each foot under the opposite knee. Let there be a comfortable gap between your feet and your pelvis. Anchor down through your hips and seat and get heavy through your lower body.
- Lift the crown of your head high to lengthen your spine.
- Place your palms down or up on your legs or take a mudra (hand position) of your choice.
- Soften your shoulders down your back and relax your facial muscles.

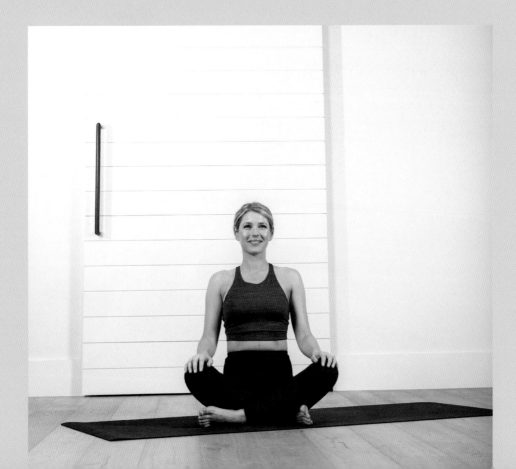

Modifications and Adaptations

- If you haven't done this pose for a while and feel discomfort, try sitting with your back against a wall or sit close to a wall and slide a yoga block between your shoulder blades and the wall for support. If you have knee pain, build your foundation of block or blankets to lift your hips higher.

- *Easy seated twist*: Grab your right knee with your left hand. Place your right fingertips behind your sacrum. Turn your chin so you look over your back shoulder. With each inhale, sit taller and stretch your spine. With each exhale, pull your belly back and twist from your core. Repeat on the left side (shown).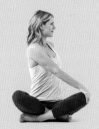

- *Easy seated fold*: Keep your ankles crossed, walk your hands forward, and bow your head and heart toward the ground. Breathe into your middle and upper back.

Thread the Needle
Parsva Balasana

Thread the needle is a twist that opens the shoulders, chest, and upper back. It is a great pose to use in an opening sequence, to reintegrate your breath after a resting pose, or to prep before backbends and binds.

Alignment

- On all fours, thread your right arm under your left armpit and rest your right cheek on the mat.

- Walk your left hand slightly forward, tent your fingers, and hug your top shoulder blade toward your spine.

- Hold, then unwind to return through tabletop pose and repeat on the other side.

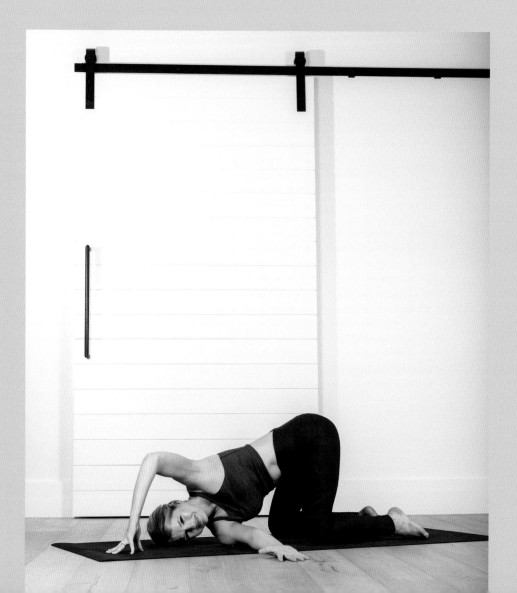

Knees-to-Chest
Apanasana

Knees-to-chest is a soothing transitional shape and counterpose that can be used throughout your practice. It creates space in the lower back and helps relieve digestive stress. It also reminds you to practice self-love as you give yourself a big hug.

Alignment

- Lie on your back and squeeze both knees into your chest.
- Wrap your arms around your shins or hold your legs behind your knees. Hug into a small ball.
- Flex your feet and awaken your toes.

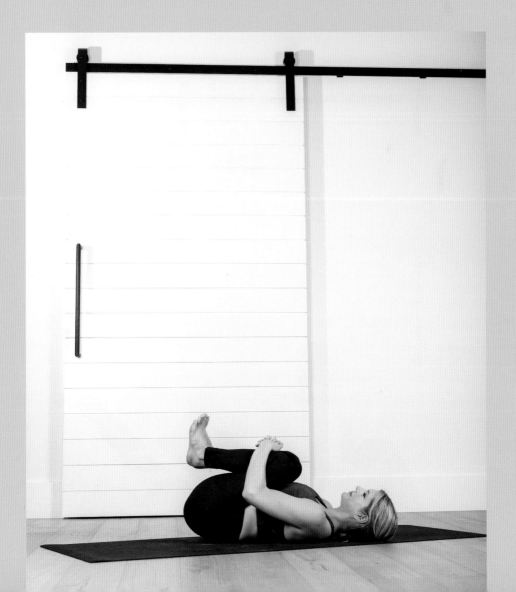

Rock 'n' Rolls

About the Pose

Rock 'n' rolls are a core-building transition. They can be used anytime during your practice and are an awakening transition as you come up from lying down.

Alignment

- Lying on your back, squeeze both knees into your chest.
- Flex your feet and awaken your toes.
- Hold your legs either behind your knees or on the fronts of your shins.
- Using your core strength, rock back and forth, from your shoulders to your toes.

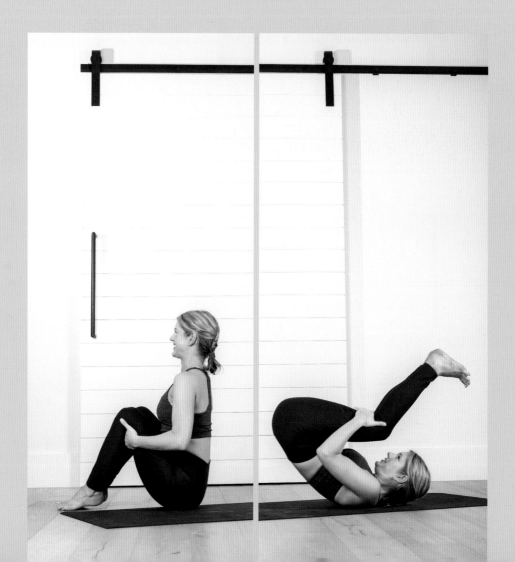

Supported Hero Pose
Virasana

About the Pose

Supported hero pose is an alternative to easy pose for seated meditation and offers many of the same grounding and calming benefits. It stretches the hips, thighs, knees, ankles, and feet; improves circulation through the entire lower body; relieves tired legs; and strengthens the feet.

Alignment

- Kneel on the floor with your shins parallel, the tops of your feet on the ground, your toes facing the back of your mat, and your heels by your hips.
- Sit on a block, cushion, or folded blanket between your heels to elevate your hips higher than your knees. Ensure that both sit bones are supported and your pelvis is neutral.
- Slide your knees together. Place your hands on your thighs, with your palms facing up or down, or use a mudra of your choice.
- Lift your shoulders to your ears and roll your shoulders down and back to open across your chest. Lengthen the tailbone toward the floor.
- Set your gaze straight ahead or close your eyes and tune in to your breath.

Modifications and Adaptations

Add as much support as you need, such as blocks or blankets, to lift your seat and empower the circulation in your legs and ensure there is no pain in your knees. You want to create a seat that is comfortable. To deepen the pose, remove the props supporting your seat and sit on the floor between your heels.

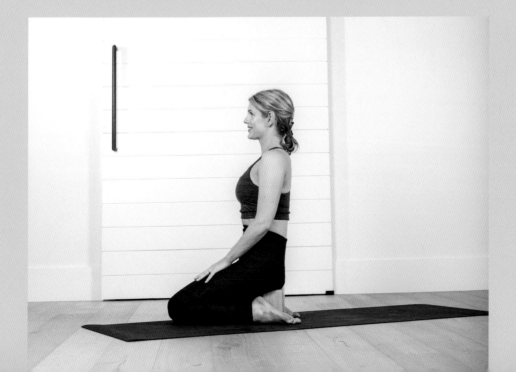

You are not creating a new you; you are releasing a hidden you. The process is one of self-discovery. The hidden you that wants to emerge is in perfect balance.

Deepak Chopra

Warm-Up Poses

Warm-up poses are full-body and dynamic postures that begin to build heat, focus, and flow. They include the poses that comprise Sun Salutations A and B, as well as variations. Warm-up poses strengthen, lengthen, flex and extend all the main muscles of the body, and when practiced in succession in these sacred sequences they distribute prana throughout your entire body as you link your movements with your breath.

Mountain Pose
Tadasasana

About the Pose

Mountain pose enlivens your body from the inside out. As you root down through your feet and legs and lift through your entire spinal column and the crown of your head, you open and light up your body and maximize the energy flowing within you. Mountain pose lengthens and opens the upper body, chest, and shoulders and counteracts the repetitive motions of life today that cause the shoulders to round forward, like being on a smartphone, sitting at a computer, or driving. In mountain pose, you train your body to stand firm in your power.

Mountain pose is the blueprint for all yoga poses. All asanas build from the foundation and optimal alignment of tadasana, so look for the structure of mountain pose within every pose of your practice.

Alignment

- Stand with your feet together at the top of your mat, with your big toes touching, and your heels slightly separated.

> continued

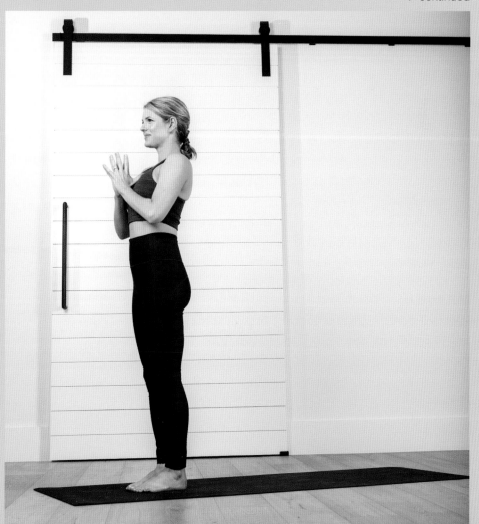

> continued

- Ground down through all four corners of both feet and extend the crown of your head toward the sky.

- Lift your kneecaps, engage your quadriceps, and hug your outer shins in toward each other.

- Lift your lower abdomen up and in, and from this lift of your core, press back down into the earth. Knit your front ribs together and in as you expand your middle back.

- With your arms alongside your body, turn your palms forward (not pictured) or place your hands at heart center (anjali mudra) by bringing your palms together at the center of your chest, which emphasizes the connectedness of your whole body and being.

- Set your gaze straight ahead so that your neck is long and neutral, or if taking anjali mudra, set your drishti at your fingertips. Steady your breath, and return to your center.

Modifications and Adaptations

Upward Salute (Urdhva Hastasana): Upward salute is a variation of mountain pose with the arms extended skyward. Dig deep roots through your feet and reach to the sky through your fingertips. Upward salute is one of the poses within traditional sun salutation A.

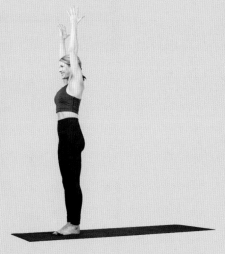

- From mountain pose, sweep both arms to the sky on your inhale, and lengthen through your entire body.

- Either separate your hands shoulder-width apart, with your palms facing one another, or unite your palms overhead.

Mountain Pose with Side Bend: This is a great variation to add to sun salutation A to create more length and opening through the side of your body and prepare you for deeper poses later in your sequence.

- Hold your left wrist with your right hand and create wisdom mudra with your left hand by connecting your thumb and your index finger. This mudra helps uplift dull energy, so use it to support you in creating more lift and length through your entire body.

- On your exhale, lean your torso to the right. Press your feet down, activate your legs, and lift into your core. Breathe space into your left ribs as you lift out of your hips and lengthen through both sides.

- Inhale and transition your torso back to center. Switch the grip of your hands.

- On your exhale, side bend to the left. Lift your lower abdomen. Activate your legs as you lift up and lengthen.

- With your inhale, return to center to upward salute. You can unite your palms to prayer overheard to accent the upward lift of your pose.

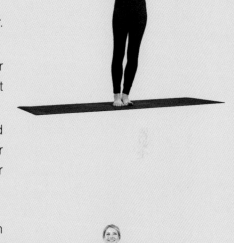

Open-Arm Twist: This standing twist is a variation of mountain pose. Adding this open-arm twists to your sun salutation will ignite your core and create opening across your chest that you can use to build into more advanced poses later in your practice.

- Extend both arms high on your inhale; use your exhale to twist. Reach your left arm forward and your right arm back. Squeeze your shoulders to your back and expand through your hands.

- With your inhale, return to center and lift both arms high.

- Exhale and twist in the other direction, reaching your right arm forward and left arm back (shown).

- Inhale and return to center, reach both arms up.

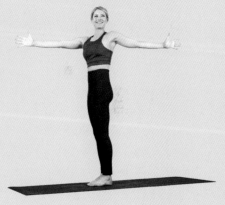

One leg tadasana: Stand in tadasana and lift one knee up to hip level, so that you are balancing on one foot. This is a transitional pose that is used in power sequences when working between standing and balancing poses.

Downward-Facing Dog
Adho Mukha Svanasana

About the Pose

We return to downward-facing dog repeatedly in power yoga, and it can be considered an active home base. Downward-facing dog gives access to power, freedom, and equanimity. It calms the nervous system, works on overall flexibility, decompresses the spine, tones the arms, sculpts the legs, and opens the shoulders. Every time you return to this pose, check in and notice how your body responds to your practice. Note that downward-facing dog is often called down dog for short.

Alignment

- Plant your hands shoulder-distance apart or wider at the top of your mat, spread your fingers, and root down through your knuckles, especially your index-finger knuckles.
- Lift your hips and straighten your legs to create an inverted V shape. Separate your feet to hip-width apart and align your feet at twelve o'clock.
- Ground down through all four corners of your feet and press your heels toward the mat. Pull your thigh bones back.
- Activate your legs and arms by firming from the skin to the muscle and into the bones.
- Let your head hang in line with your arms. Set your drishti between your ankles.

Modifications and Adaptations

Your weight should be equally distributed between your hands and your feet, so you may need to widen or shorten your base, depending on your needs. When your stance is too short, down dog can feel tight and constrained, especially through the shoulders, lower back, and wrists. Open your base and widen your hands and feet to access more power, freedom, and equanimity.

If you notice your lower back rounding, try bending your knees to help lengthen your back. You can always come down to all fours (tabletop) or take child's pose if you need to modify your down dog or base pose.

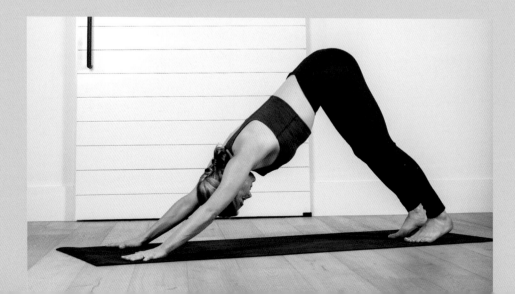

Down Dog Splits

About the Pose

Down dog splits, sometimes known as three-legged dog, is a modern variation of downward-facing dog. It emphasizes rooting through your foundation and lengthening from your base to the sky. This pose is frequently added to sun salutation variations or integrated into creative sequences to highlight extension on an inhale.

Alignment

- From downward-facing dog, on your inhale, lift your right leg high. Lift from your inner right thigh, keep both hip bones squared to the earth, and ensure all five toes face the ground.

- Move from core strength rather than from the periphery. Lengthen from your right wrist through your right heel.

- Repeat on the other side and hold for the same count or add a flow sequence for one inhale.

Modifications and Adaptations

To increase side body and quad stretch, bend your top knee and stack your hips. Keep the equanimity in your shoulders as you add the twist of your pelvis.

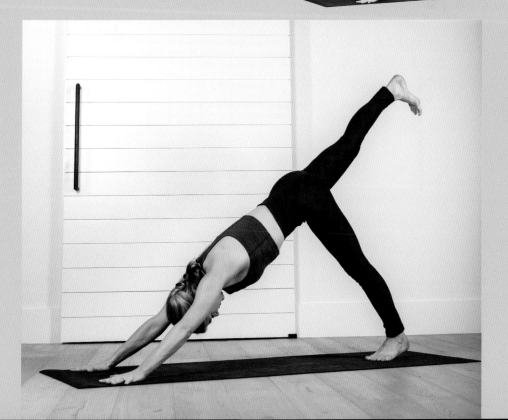

Halfway Lift
Ardha Uttanasana

About the Pose

Halfway lift creates length in the front body before folding forward. It stretches the hamstring and lower back. It tones and strengthens the back and abdominal muscles, improving overall posture.

Alignment

- From standing forward fold, bend your knees, slide your palms to your shins, and press firmly into your legs.
- Lengthen the crown of your head forward, extend your tailbone back, and align your torso parallel to the mat.
- Pull your shoulder blades onto your back and broaden across your chest.
- Set your gaze to the ground, so your neck is neutral and aligned with your entire spine.

Modifications and Adaptations

Bend your knees as much as you need to maintain a flat back. If your back or shoulders start to round, bend your knees more.

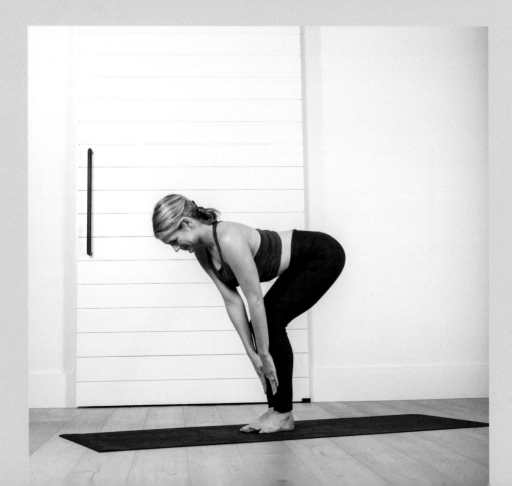

Standing Forward Fold
Uttanasana

About the Pose

Standing forward fold unwinds the hamstrings, calves, and lower back. All forward folds and inversions help infuse the brain with fresh energy and oxygen, which soothes and revitalizes the nervous system, calms the brain, and helps relieve stress. As you release your head and the muscles in your neck, you unravel tension in the upper back and neck and open the pathway to bring more oxygen-rich blood into the brain. The folding action stimulates and strengthens the digestive organs. Standing forward fold done while holding the opposite elbows and keeping your knees softly bent is often called ragdoll. If you notice you are rigid or tight in this fold, bend your knees more and allow yourself to be both rooted and spacious and mirror the energy of a flexible ragdoll.

> continued

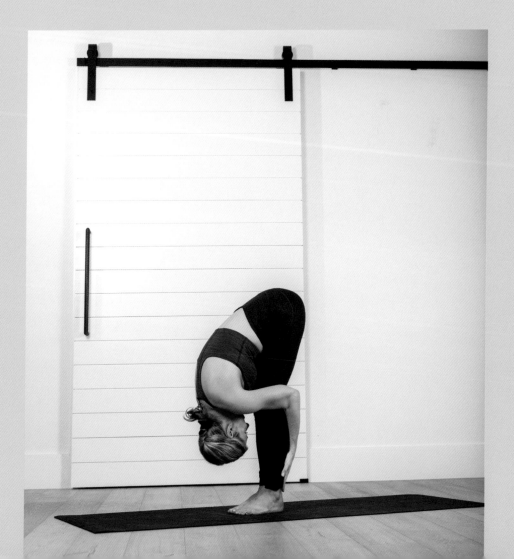

> *continued*

Alignment

- Either stand with your feet together or separate your feet so they are below your hips and parallel to each other. Press down through all four corners of your feet.

- Hinge at your hips, fold your torso over your thighs, and release the crown of your head toward the ground. Touch your front ribs to your thighs. Bend your knees as much as you need to lengthen your lower back. Rotate your inner thighs back. Tilt your hips toward the sky and stack them over the tops of your heels. Engage your quadriceps and lift your lower abdomen.

- Create the hand placement that feels best to you. You can grab opposite elbows, keep your fingertips on the ground, or interlace your fingers into a bind at your lower back.

- Relax your head and let your neck lengthen. Lift your breath to fill the space between your ribs. Massage your back body with healing, balanced breath.

Modifications and Adaptations

Bending your knees helps lengthen the lower back and get deeper into the muscles of the legs. For more balance and support, you can place your fingertips on blocks by your feet.

High Plank
Utthita Chaturanga Dandasana

About the Pose

High plank is an igniting posture that generates presence, focus, and heat and builds an inner fire. It builds upper- and lower-body strength and creates total body integration. High plank is one of the poses in sun salutations and the vinyasa (see page 98). It can be used by itself for core strengthening and intensified through variations.

Alignment

- From downward-facing dog, shift forward and stack your shoulders over your wrists and extend your heels to the back of your mat in a high push-up pose.

- Lengthen your crown forward and reach your heels back.

- Firmly press your knuckles into your mat and soften your thoracic spine (upper and middle back).

- Hug your thumbs toward the center of your mat and broaden across your collarbones.

- Lengthen your tailbone toward your heels and lift your lower belly up and in. Activate your breath.

> continued

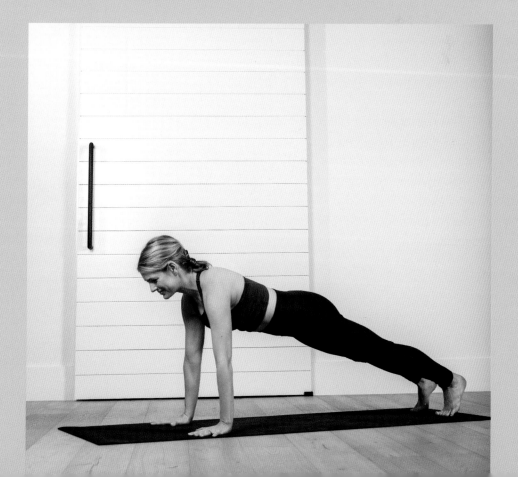

> *continued*

Modifications and Adaptations

- To reduce the intensity of plank, bring your knees down to the mat or come into tabletop pose (page 64).

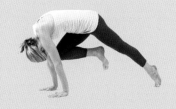

- *Plank curl or knee-to-nose*: In plank pose, on an exhale, lift your right foot and curl your right knee in toward your nose. Keep your shoulders stacked over your wrists and arch your upper back. Pull your heel up, lift your lower abdomen, and squeeze into your center. You can hold for multiple breaths to build heat and core strength, or tap either triceps for variation. Extend back to plank or down dog splits on an inhale.

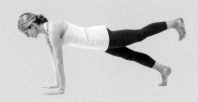

- *Three-point plank*: From plank pose, lift one foot off the earth, with your heel in line with your hip. Press your heel toward the wall behind you, flex your foot, and pull your toes toward your chest. Engage your leg muscles to the bones and pull your thigh bone into your hip socket. Hold for 5 heating breaths or use as a transition. Repeat on the other side.

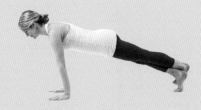

- *Plank with ankles crossed*: Lift one leg to hip level and flex your lifted foot. Cross your lifted ankle over your bottom ankle. Engage your legs together. This connection and hugging energy generates power. Press your heels back, lengthen your crown forward, and lift your lower abdomen.

Low Plank

Chaturanga Dandasana

About the Pose

Chaturanga, or low plank, encourages full-body integration and the coordination of your entire body.

Alignment

- In plank, press into the first two knuckles (thumb and index finger) of each hand, with your palms flat.

- Look forward past the top of your mat and press to your toes. With your exhale, lower halfway down, hovering your shoulders at elbow height.

- Your elbows should form a 90-degree angle. Pull your arm bones on your back and open across your chest.

- Engage your lower abdomen and tighten your legs so that your weight is distributed through your entire form.

- Press your tailbone toward your heels.

Modifications and Adaptations

To modify and build healthy alignment and strength, bring your knees down to the mat. Shoulders often round forward and collapse in chaturanga, and the bottom goes up. This disintegrates the upper and lower halves of the body, you lose power, and it puts tremendous pressure on the shoulders and rotator cuff. With your knees down to the mat, keep your chest broad and open and your sides long. Lengthen your tailbone down and lift your low belly up and in. With your whole body working as a unit, lower to a modified chaturanga, bending your elbows to about 90 degrees. You can also lower your whole body to the mat and transition to low cobra rather than upward-facing dog.

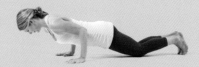

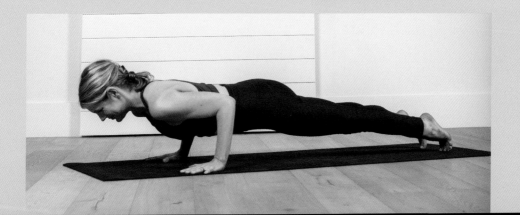

Upward-Facing Dog
Urdhva Mukha Svanasana

About the Pose

Upward-facing dog is an active backbend within the vinyasa that opens the entire front body; tones the muscles of the arms, shoulders, and back; and engages the legs. It opens the chest, which expands your ability to breathe more deeply and embody flow.

Alignment

- Start by lying down on your front body. Press your palms into the mat and slide your thumbs back by your lower ribs, so that your elbows stack over your wrists. Place your feet hip-width apart and press down into the tops of your feet. Within the vinyasa you'll move from low plank (chaturanga) to upward-facing dog.

- Root down through the triads of your hands, straighten your arms to press the earth away from you and stack your shoulders over your wrists.

- Draw your upper arms back and lift and open across your chest. Engage your quadriceps and abdomen, and lift your thighs off the ground.

- Set your gaze straight ahead so that your chin is neutral or lift your gaze to the sky.

Modifications and Adaptations

If your shoulders are rounding forward or your thighs are on the ground, upward-facing dog can feel tight and constricted rather than open and expansive. To modify, push down through your knuckles, bend your elbows, and pull your upper arm bones onto your back, and broaden across your chest. Press the tops of your feet down, hug your outer shins in, and lift your thighs off the mat. Then press your hands down, straighten your arms, and lift your gaze.

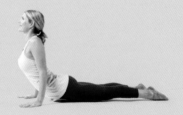

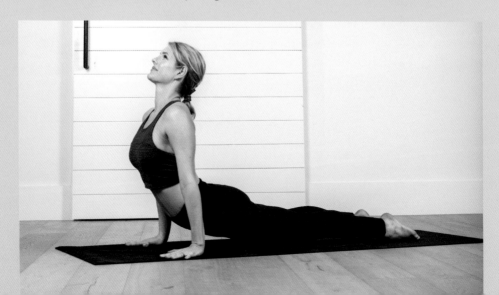

Low Cobra
Bhujangasana

About the Pose

Low cobra helps strengthen the muscles of the back and build the body awareness needed for upward-facing dog. If your thighs are resting on the ground in up dog, low cobra is a great modification to create healthy alignment for the lower back and shoulders as you move through the many vinyasas in the power yoga practice.

Alignment

- From high plank, lower your whole front body down to the mat.
- Untuck your toes and press down through the tops of your feet and toenails and firm your leg muscles.
- Slide your palms back so that your thumbs are in line with your lowest ribs.
- As you inhale, engage your back body and curl your chest up.
- Keep your gaze down at your mat and your neck neutral.

Modifications and Adaptations

To modify and increase the strength of your upper back, lift your palms off the ground and hug your shoulder blades in toward your spine.

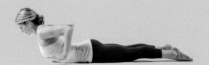

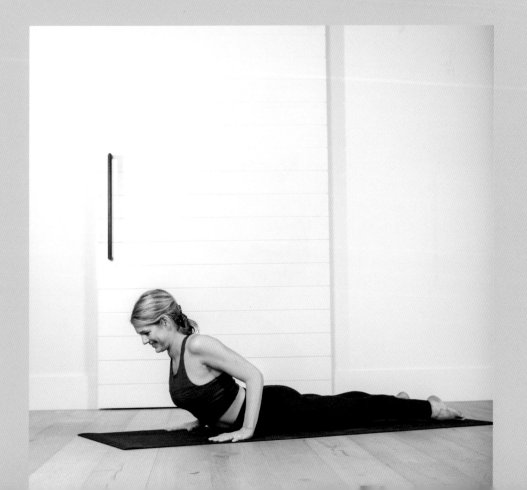

Chair Pose
Utkatasana

About the Pose

Chair pose builds inner heat and stamina because it sculpts the muscles of the legs and butt. It stimulates your metabolism and circulation and increases your heart rate. Chair pose is powerful and teaches us to relax into intensity and meet stress with steady, full breath.

Alignment

- From a standing forward fold, bring your feet together, with your big toes touching at the center of your mat. Bend your knees deeply as if you were sitting in a chair.
- Stay grounded through all four corners of your feet. On an inhale, lift your chest and arms toward the sky.
- Separate your hands at shoulder-width apart and slightly rotate your pinky fingers in toward each other to broaden your upper back. Relax your shoulders down.
- Set your gaze straight ahead. As the heat builds in your legs, continue to generate your steady and balanced breath.

Modifications and Adaptations

To add more leg and core strengthening, you can squeeze a block between your thighs and hug into your centerline.

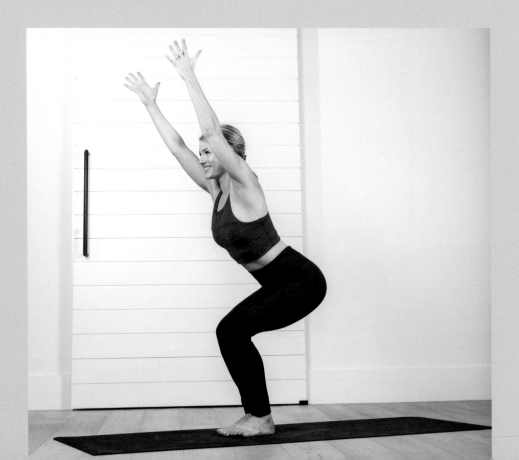

Warrior I
Virabhadrasana I

About the Pose

This dynamic pose creates total body integration and activation. It strengthens the legs, opens the hips, and prepares the entire body for the rest of your practice. Warrior I is an opportunity to embody what you stand for in your life. Take up your space and breathe in your purpose and power.

Alignment

- From downward-facing dog, at the base of your exhale, use your core strength to step your right foot to your right thumb.

- Dial your left heel down to the mat, and seal the outer edge of your foot to the ground. Hug your heels toward one another to ignite your legs. Inhale and lift your chest and your arms overhead.

- Keep a deep bend in your front knee and stack your knee over your front ankle.

- From your hips, ground down through your feet.

> continued

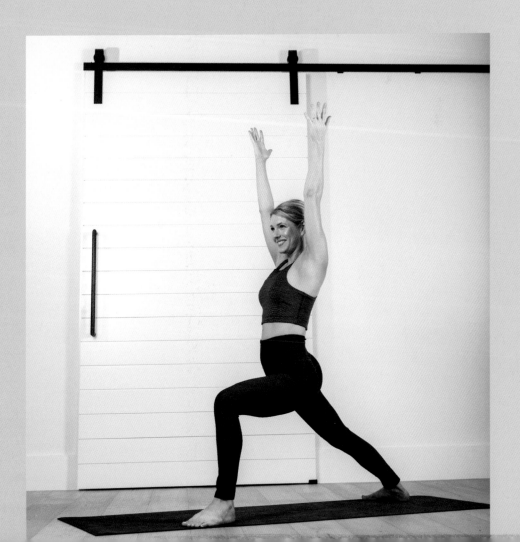

> *continued*

- Work to square both hip bones and your ribs forward. Lower your tailbone and lift your low belly up and in.

- From your waist, stretch up and out through your fingertips.

- Breathe deeply as you embody your power in this dynamic pose. Repeat on the other side.

Modifications and Adaptations

- Explore the angle of your back foot that works best for you. Try aiming your toes to the outer edge of your mat and create a 90-degree angle and notice how that feels. Now try 60 degrees and 45 degrees. Where do you feel most connection and power with your back leg? Use the position that feels most powerful to you.

- If your hips feel tight, try increasing the distance between your heels toward the outer edges of your mat. Going wider can give you more access to more rotation and allow you to square your hips forward. Remember, the alignment cues are guides for you to create a pose where you feel most powerful.

Opening Sequences

The opening sequence can be one pose or a few simple poses linked together. The opening sequence serves to further connect you with your breath as you gently coax the body open by adding simple movements. Each group of poses can be used in sequence at the beginning of your practice as you center yourself and prepare your body and mind. These postures are not only reserved for the start of class. You can also integrate them into other parts of your practice or return to them to rest and recharge. In any sequence, you will always do the poses on the right side, and then repeat on your left side. The opening sequence is sealed by coming to the top of the mat in mountain pose, with your hands at heart center. This is an opportunity to pause, set your intention for your practice, and honor the connection with all of life by chanting om.

OM

Om is said to be the sound of the universe. It is a symbol of our connection to all living beings and is the current of life that runs through it all. It's also a way to mark the beginning and end of yoga classes. Chanting om can be intimidating to newer students, and you are by no means required to participate. It can also be liberating as you allow yourself to let your voice be heard and connect to others.

The sound of om has three parts. They represent the past, present, and future as well as the body, mind, and spirit. These are the three sounds:

1. Ah
2. Oh
3. Mm

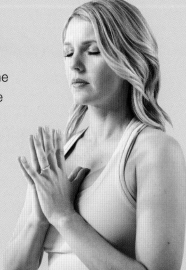

When you chant om, press the palms together at the center of the chest, your thumb touching your breastbone (see figure 4.1). This hand placement is known as anjali mudra. You can close your eyes or set your soft vision at your fingertips. This ritual of hand placement, focus, and chanting harnesses your energy and brings everyone together to start and end the class.

Try chanting om each time you practice during your 28-day power yoga plan. Notice what part of your om is the most powerful and how you feel after you use your voice to help kick-off your practice. As you practice this simple and powerful chant at home,

Figure 4.1 Hand placement for om.

you'll tap into more confidence and clarity with your voice. You can carry this into your practice at a yoga studio or harness the energy of your voice in other areas of your life.

Your opening sequence can introduce subtle shapes and motions that you will weave through your whole practice. As you begin, mindfully create this union of your body and breath and gently awaken your body before the sun salutations and dynamic sequences. The opening of your practice is not the time to rush or force anything. To get the most out of your whole practice, its essential to ignite your body-mind connection as you begin; otherwise, yoga can become just become another thing you mark off on your to-do list. Your body and breath working as one makes this practice mindful and generates presence.

Use the opening sequences to come out of your head and into your body. Take as much time as you need to allow yourself to integrate mind, body, and spirit. I recommend 1 to 5 minutes in the opening pose and another 10 breaths or more in each pose of the opening sequence. These sequences are guides, so modify them as you need to and as time allows.

Sample Opening Sequence 1

This opening sequence will help you focus on your foundation.

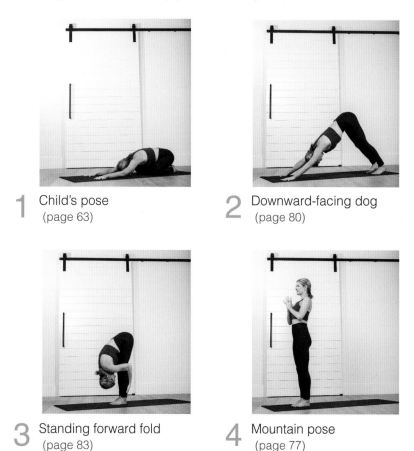

1 Child's pose
(page 63)

2 Downward-facing dog
(page 80)

3 Standing forward fold
(page 83)

4 Mountain pose
(page 77)

Sample Opening Sequence 2

This opening sequence will help you relax the muscles of your back and neck as you start to unwind your spine.

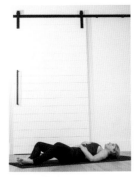

1 Reclined bound angle
(page 68)

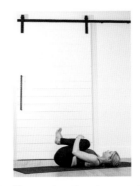

2 Knees-to-chest
(page 73)

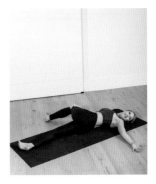

3 Supine twist
(page 69)

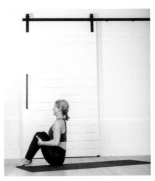

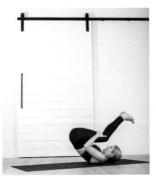

4 Rock' n' rolls
(page 74)

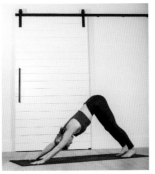

5 Downward-facing dog
(page 80)

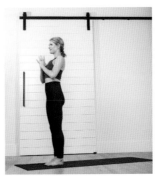

6 Mountain pose
(page 77)

Sample Opening Sequence 3

In this opening sequence, you will sit in stillness to help you anchor into your breath and body and begin to lengthen and release the muscles along your spine.

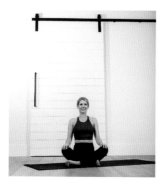

1 Easy pose
(page 70)

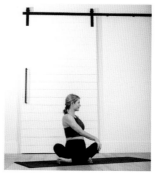

2 Easy seated twist
(page 71)

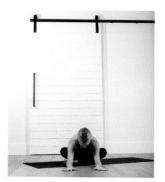

3 Easy seated fold
(page 71)

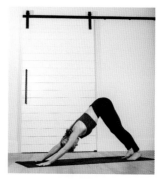

4 Downward-facing dog
(page 80)

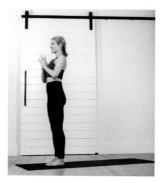

5 Mountain pose
(page 77)

Sample Opening Sequence 4

This opening sequence connects you to the deep tissues and sensations in your hips and legs.

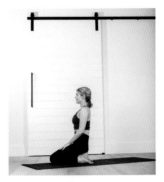

1 Supported hero pose
(page 75)

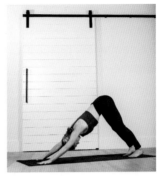

2 Downward-facing dog
(page 80)

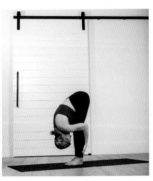

3 Standing forward fold or ragdoll
(page 83)

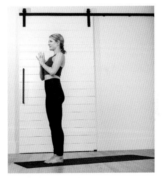

4 Mountain pose
(page 77)

Vinyasa

Vinyasa means "flow" and is the linking of breath with movement. In classes, it's commonly used to describe the connection of one pose to the next, as within sun salutations or in a sequence as you transition from one side to the other. You'll often hear teachers say "vinyasa" to transition to the other side as they guide you in building a sequence. It's the shorthand term for low plank to upward-facing dog to downward-facing dog.

Energetically, a vinyasa wipes the slate clean as you begin again on the second side of your sequence or move on to the next element of your practice. You can always leave out the vinyasa or adapt the poses to meet your needs. For example, to lessen the intensity of your practice, you could leave out low plank. To increase the heat, you could add multiple push-ups.

In the pose descriptions and sequences throughout this book, I'll lead you through the cues on your first side. Then you can choose to take a vinyasa and build the same pose or sequence on the other side. In power yoga, we repeat the vinyasa—the flow from chaturanga on your exhale, to up dog on your inhale, to down dog on your exhale—again and again throughout the practice. Use your entire breath to complete each pose, and never rush through your vinyasa. The simple sequence of repetitive poses, when practiced with optimal alignment and breath, deliver power, coordination, and strength.

Let's take a deeper look at the poses that comprise the vinyasa.

Vinyasa

1 Exhale: chaturanga.

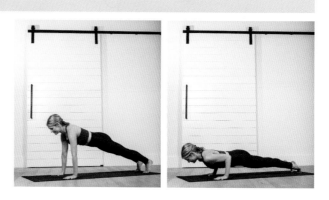

Chaturanga is the movement from high plank to low plank. From plank pose, press forward on your tiptoes and shift your shoulders beyond your wrists. This forward action before you lower down into the low push-up will keep your shoulders and lower back open. Lengthen your tailbone toward your heels and engage your core as you shift forward to your toes to integrate your upper- and lower-body. Look forward, not down, to help keep your chest and shoulders open. Look with your eyes, rather than lifting your whole head. Lower your shoulders to 90 degrees, but don't dip your shoulders lower than your elbows. The lower you go, the more effort it takes to press into upward dog. Keep your neck long and in line with the rest of your spine. If you need to modify these poses, drop your knees to the ground to create a modified plank, or when lowering into the low push-up, go all the way down to the ground, bringing your belly and chest to the mat.

2 Inhale: upward-facing dog.

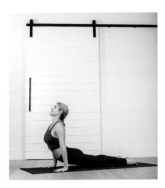

Pull your shoulder blades in toward your spine and down your back, and lift your sternum skyward to open your chest and maximize your breath. In up dog, your hands and the tops of your feet are your foundation. Everything else, including your thighs, is engaged and lifting away from your mat. If you need to modify, lower all the way down to the ground and do low cobra (see p. 89), rooting down through the tops of your feet and lifting your chest on your inhale. You can lift your palms as well to build upper-back strength.

3 Exhale: downward-facing dog.

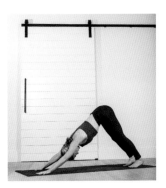

Lift your hips up and back to down dog. The movement is initiated from your core, your center. Either transition to the soles of both feet simultaneously or one foot at a time. Ground down through your toe mounds and heels. Press your thighs back. Let your head follow the rest of your body and land your drishti between your heels. If you need to modify this pose, press back through child's pose and then up to your downward-facing dog.

Sun Salutations

Sun salutations are the warm-up and building blocks to every power yoga practice. They follow the opening pose and opening sequence, after the om. The vinyasa is rooted within both sun salutation A and B. These foundational and dynamic sequences are performed at the pace of the breath in a flow—one breath, one movement. They use the whole body; get the heart pumping; boost circulation; begin to open and awaken the entire body, including all the major joints; and prepare the body for the entire practice.

Traditionally, yogis used the ritual of the physical practice (asana) in the early morning to harness the power of the sun and greet the new day. The sun gives energy to all life as it lights the earth. The movements within sun salutations (surya namaskar) are designed to awaken energy at the navel center, a major energetic center, and radiate that energy through your entire body. Sun salutations cultivate an inward focus while stoking your inner fire and building a cleansing heat. These activating sequences will plug you right into your breath and into the power of renewal that is available by linking the body, breath, and attention.

You can do a few minutes of sun salutations as your daily morning practice, add them into longer practices, or do one at a time when you need a little boost. In traditional ashtanga vinyasa yoga, you do five sun salutation A's and five sun salutation B's with five breaths between them in downward-facing dog. In your power yoga practice, you can modify these sequences depending on your goals and the time constraints of each practice. However, I recommend always including sun salutations A and B as part of your practice. Remember the wisdom within the tradition of yoga and use the blueprint of sun salutations to open and awaken your body before your go deeper into your practice.

Sun Salutation A

Start by standing at the top of your mat with your feet together and bring your palms to connect at the center of your chest. Press all four corners of your feet into the ground, firm your leg muscles, and lift your lower abdomen up and in. From this lift of your core, press back down into the earth, and feel the muscles from your core to your toes engage. Feel the rooting of your legs and lift your chest toward the sky, and the power start to awaken within your body.

Take a few deep breaths in and out of your nose and start to build your ujjayi breath. Aim to balance the pace and flow of your inhale and exhale. Before you begin moving, close your eyes and take a moment to set an intention for your practice. As you declare your energetic aim, every breath and movement becomes infused with this purpose. Keep your breath flowing through your nose as you move through sun salutation A.

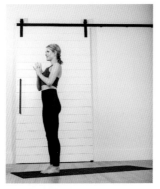

1 Mountain pose, with hands at heart center.

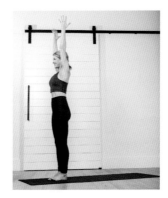

2 Inhale: upward salute.

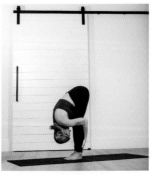

3 Exhale: standing forward fold.

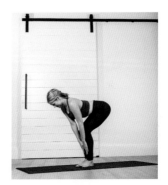

4 Inhale: halfway lift.

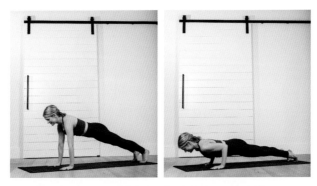

5 Exhale: chaturanga (high plank to low plank).

> continued

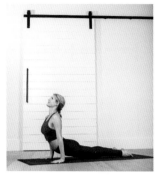

6 Inhale: upward-facing dog.

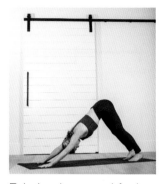

7 Exhale: downward-facing dog; hold for 5 breaths.

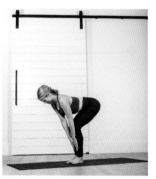

8 After your fifth exhale, step or jump to the top of your mat. Inhale: halfway lift.

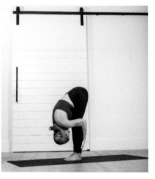

9 Exhale: standing forward fold.

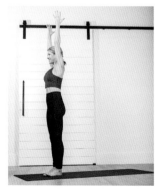

10 Inhale: upward salute.

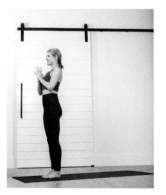

11 Exhale: mountain pose, with hands at heart center.

When you feel complete with your practice of sun salutation A, pause with your hands in prayer at heart center (anjali mudra), close your eyes, and take a few deep breaths. If you set an intention, bring it to the forefront of your mind and let the energy of your intention guide you into the rest of your practice.

Sun Salutation B

After sun salutation A, continue with sun salutation B as follows:

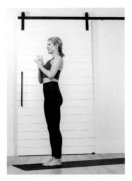

1 Mountain pose, with arms by your sides or hands at heart center.

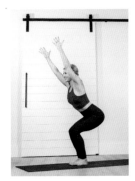

2 Inhale: chair pose.

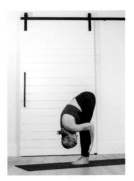

3 Exhale: standing forward fold.

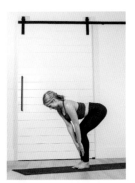

4 Inhale: halfway lift.

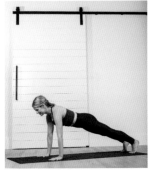

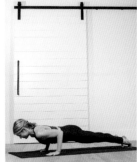

5 Exhale: chaturanga (high plank to low plank).

> continued

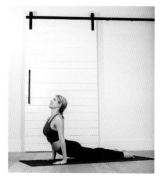

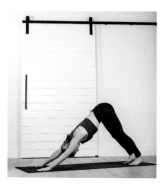

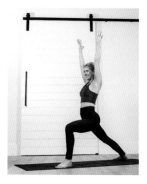

6 Inhale: upward-facing dog.

7 Exhale: downward-facing dog. At the base of your exhale; step your right foot forward.

8 Inhale: warrior I.

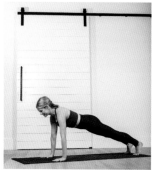

9 Exhale: chaturanga (high plank to low plank).

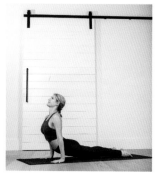

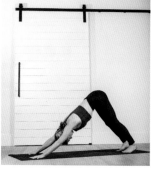

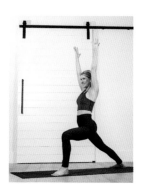

10 Inhale: upward-facing dog.

11 Exhale: downward-facing dog. At the base of your exhale; step your left foot forward.

12 Inhale: warrior I.

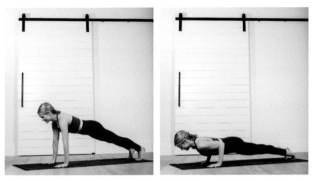

13 Exhale: chaturanga (high plank to low plank).

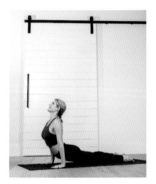

14 Inhale: upward-facing dog.

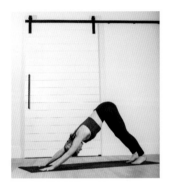

15 Exhale: downward-facing dog; hold for 5 breaths.

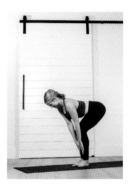

16 After your fifth exhale, step or jump to the top of your mat. Inhale: halfway lift.

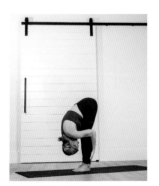

17 Exhale: standing forward fold.

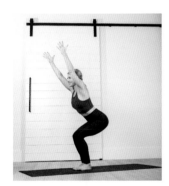

18 Inhale: chair pose.

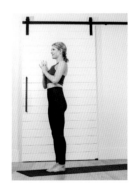

19 Exhale: mountain pose, with hands at heart center.

Sun Salutation Variations

Simple variations of sun salutation can help open the body and prepare for poses later in your sequence, like heart-opening backbends, deep twists, and binds. You'll work from the same traditional sun salutation A and B blueprints while adding poses that continue to emphasize opening on the inhale and contraction with the exhale, and prepare your body for your whole practice.

Sun Salutation A   Optional Variations

At the top of your mat, with your hands at heart center in mountain pose, add these simple variations:

Open-Arm Twists

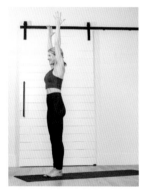 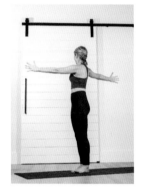 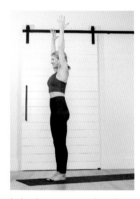

1 Inhale: upward salute.

2 Exhale: Open and twist to the right and extend your left arm forward and right arm back.

3 Inhale: upward salute.

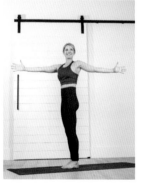 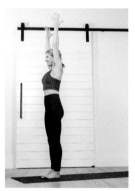 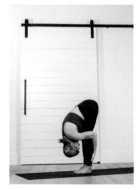

4 Exhale: Open and twist to the left on an exhale and reach your right arm forward and left arm back.

5 Inhale: upward salute.

6 Exhale: standing forward fold.

Cactus Arms

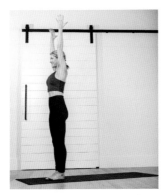

1 Inhale: upward salute.

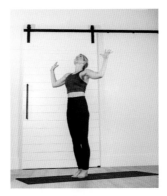

2 Exhale: Bend your elbows to 90 degrees into cactus arms by hugging your shoulder blades together and lift your chest toward the sky.

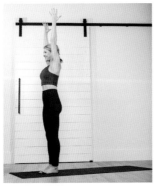

3 Inhale: upward salute.

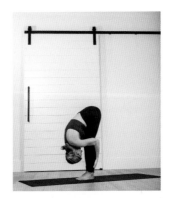

4 Exhale: standing forward fold.

> continued

Side Bends

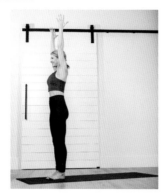

1 Inhale: upward salute.

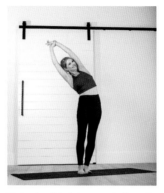

2 Exhale: Hold your left wrist with your right hand and lean to the right into a side bend.

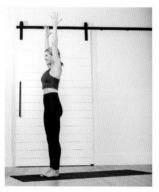

3 Inhale: upward salute.

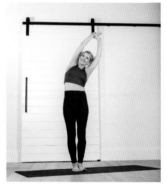

4 Exhale: Hold your right wrist with your left hand and lean to the left into a side bend.

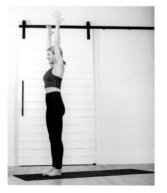

5 Inhale: upward salute.

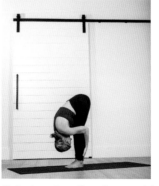

6 Exhale: standing forward fold.

Sun Salutation B   Optional Variations

These sequences build from sun salutation B and integrate other poses for more opening, heat building, and variation.

Chair Twist

From chair pose in sun salutation B, you can add twists as follows:

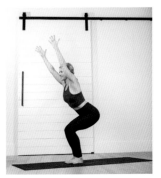

1 Inhale: chair pose.

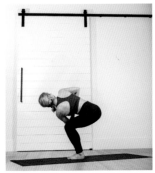

2 Exhale: Twist to the right (option to hold for one whole breath cycle).

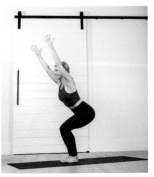

3 Inhale: chair pose.

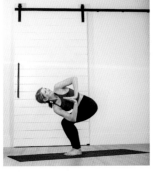

4 Exhale: Twist to the left (option to hold for one whole breath cycle).

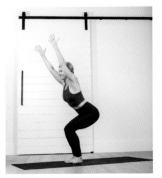

5 Inhale: chair pose.

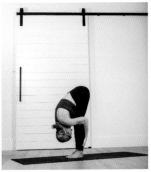

6 Exhale: standing forward fold.

> continued

Humble Warrior

From downward-facing dog in sun Salutation B, you can add humble warrior as follows (repeat on both sides):

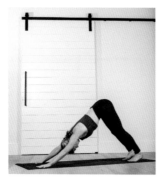

1 Exhale: downward-facing dog.

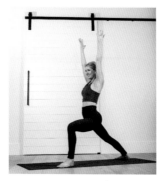

2 Inhale: warrior I (right side).

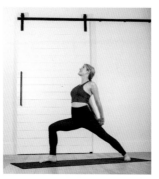

3 Exhale: Warrior I with a bind. Interlace your fingers at your lower back to create a bind. Pull your shoulder blades toward your spine.

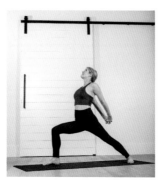

4 Inhale: Warrior I with a bind. Expand into your bind, lift your chest, and gaze up.

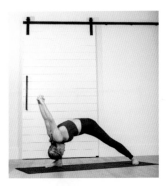 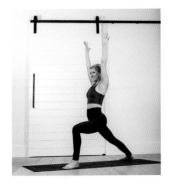

5 Exhale: Bow into humble warrior. Lower your chest and head toward the floor, and hug your right shoulder to the inside of your right knee.

6 Inhale: Warrior I (right side) and release your bind, and sweep your arms to the sky.

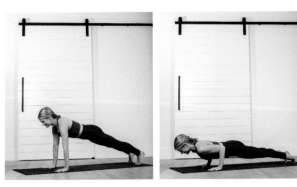

7 Exhale: move through the vinyasa and repeat on the other side.

> continued

Plank Curls

From downward-facing dog in sun salutation B, you can add one or more plank curls as follows (repeat on both sides):

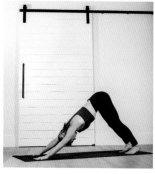

1 Exhale: downward-facing dog.

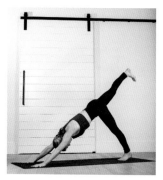

2 Inhale: down dog splits (right side).

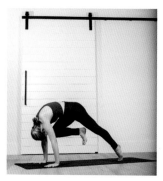

3 Exhale: Stack your shoulders over your wrists and draw your right knee to your nose for a plank curl.

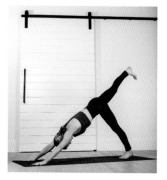

4 Inhale: down dog splits (right side).

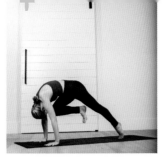 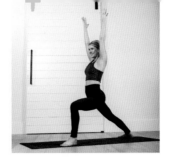

5 Exhale: Stack your shoulders over your wrists, draw your right knee to your nose for a plank curl, and then step your right foot to your right thumb.

6 Inhale: warrior I (right side).

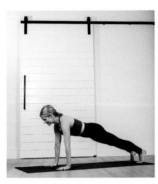 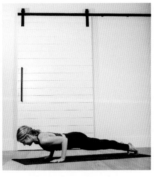

7 Exhale: move through the vinyasa and repeat on the other side.

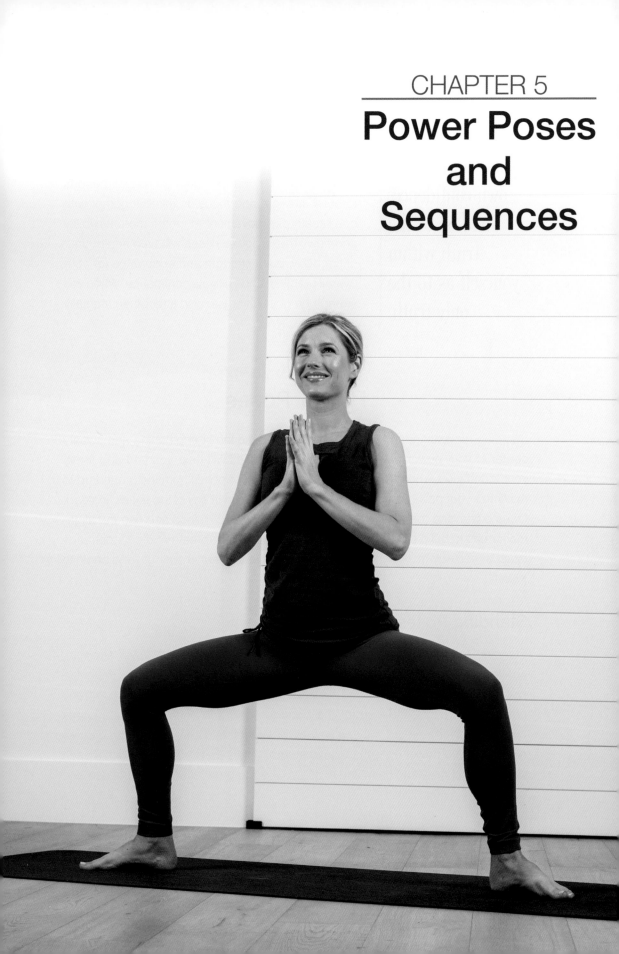

CHAPTER 5

Power Poses and Sequences

> Be a lamp to yourself. Be your own confidence. Hold on to the truth within yourself as to the only truth.
>
> Buddha

The poses and sequences within this chapter create the deeply physical center of the power yoga practice. These postures are challenging and designed to train you to find the edge and ease of every pose. They can be held for longer periods to build strength and focus or linked together with one breath per movement to create more flexibility and flow. These power poses will help sculpt your entire body, build strength and endurance for your overall practice, and cultivate confidence. When you strengthen physically, you also strengthen mentally and spiritually.

Power Poses

Standing, balancing, and twisting poses comprise the strengthening and sweaty center of your power practice. These power poses will help you find and fortify your foundation, where every pose starts. Work your poses from the ground up to maximize your power. It doesn't matter how far you go in any of the poses; instead, focus on igniting the power principles within your experience and use the alignment cues to build poses that work for you. Keep your breath and concentration intact as you add more dynamic movement, increase your challenge, and begin to sweat.

Standing Poses

Standing poses are essential to this practice because they build power, strength, and focus. Standing poses are dynamic and get energy flowing to work the entire body. They increase strength and stamina in the legs, hips, core, and back, thereby creating a strong foundation for the body to open and energize. These poses can be held for a breath within a flow or for several minutes, depending on your needs. As you power up with these postures, gently meet your edge within each pose with curiosity and calm and watch your edge grow as you stay focused and breathe.

Warrior II
Virabhadrasana II

About the Pose

Warrior II creates dynamic expansion through the whole body and increases stamina. It strengthens and stretches the legs and ankles and opens the chest, lungs, and shoulders. Warrior II creates focus and teaches you how to hone your power and concentration, and how to powerfully fill your space

Alignment

- From downward-facing dog, step your right foot forward to the top of the mat and ground your back heel to the earth.

- Press the outer edge of your back foot into the mat and lift your arch, and bend your front knee at a 90-degree angle.

- Draw your heels toward one another to ignite your inner thighs.

- With your inhale, lift up and turn open to the left side of your mat. Spread your arms wide and stack your wrists over your ankles.

> continued

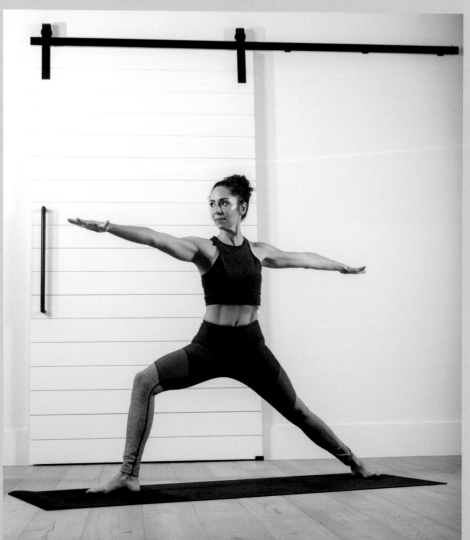

> *continued*

- Lengthen your tailbone toward the ground and engage your core.
- Spread your fingers and set your gaze over your front middle finger. Feel your body light up with life force as you concentrate.

Modifications and Adaptations

Reverse warrior. With your right foot forward, flip your front palm, reach your right arm to the sky, and slide your left arm down your back leg. Stay low and rooted through your warrior II legs, with your front knee bent at 90 degrees. Lift your chest away from your pelvis and lengthen through both side ribs. Your gaze can be up to your top hand, down at your back foot, or neutral—whatever feels best for you. Reverse warrior is a great transitional pose within a flow or a strengthening pose when held for 5 or more breaths.

Extended Side Angle
Utthita Parsvakonasana

About the Pose

This full-body power pose creates total body integration and expansion. It opens, stretches, and strengthens the legs, groin, spine, waist, chest, and shoulders while cultivating overall balance and coordination.

Alignment

- Align your heels in your wide warrior II stance. Press the outer edge of your back foot down and lift your arch.
- Keep your front knee bent, with your front femur parallel with the mat.
- Pull your front heel to the back of your mat, to ignite your inner thighs.
- Tilt your tailbone down toward your back heel and lift your belly.
- Either place your lower forearm to your thigh or place your lower hand to the outside of your front foot and press into your fingertips. Sweep your top arm overhead and lengthen the side of your body from your back heel to your fingertips.

> continued

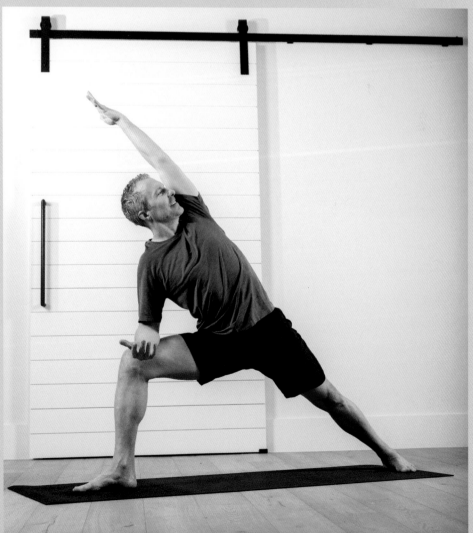

> continued

- Turn your gaze up over your top shoulder or look down to your front foot. Keep your heels, hips, and head in one plane.

- On your inhales, reach and expand from your back heel through your top hand, and on your exhales, engage your core and twist your chest more toward the sky.

Modifications and Adaptations

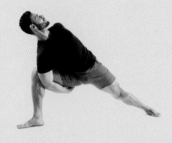

- *Extended side angle with a bind*: A bind will help to deepen the pose and open more across the chest and shoulders. Wrap your top arm behind your back and your front arm under your front leg. Interlock your fingers, draw your shoulder blades together, and lift and lengthen your chest forward. For a half bind, wrap your top arm behind your back and reach for your inner thigh of your front leg.

Triangle
Utthita Trikonasana

About the Pose

Triangle is an expansive pose that enlivens the whole body as you stretch in all directions. It requires deep roots through your legs to lift into your center and cultivate abdominal strength. It strengthens the vital organs and stimulates digestion. Triangle pose stretches and strengthens the legs and ankles, while opening the shoulders, chest, and spine.

Alignment

- Take a wide warrior stance on your mat. Turn your front foot to twelve o'clock. Align your heels and seal the outer edges of both feet to the ground.

- Straighten both legs while keeping a slight bend at your front knee. From your hips to your heels, root down to create a solid foundation to the earth. Lift the energy up your legs, hug your muscles to the bones, and draw your energy into your core.

> continued

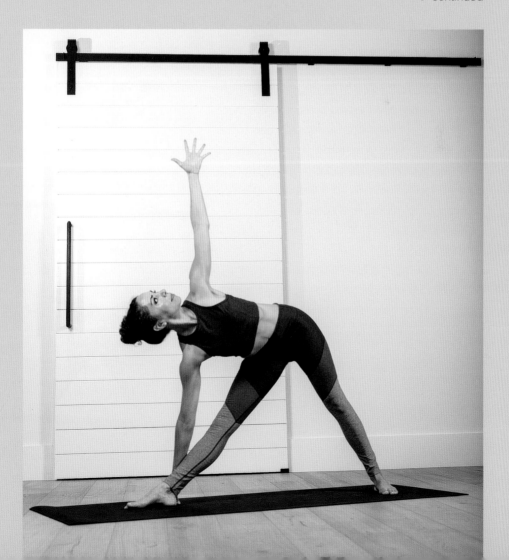

> *continued*

- Spread your arms wide and align your wrists over your ankles. Hinge forward and reach your front hand toward the top of your mat. When you can't lengthen anymore, place your front hand to the outside of your front foot and press into your fingertips. Reach your top arm to the sky. Open across your chest and make one line from your lower hand through your top fingertips.

- Knit your front ribs together, engage your core, and twist your chest high with every exhale.

- Lift your gaze to your top hand, look down at your front foot, or find a neutral gaze in between. Do whatever feels best to you.

Modifications and Adaptations

- If it doesn't feel good to have your front hand on the floor, your chest is turning toward the ground, or you are crunching through your side ribs, support your bottom hand or fingertips on a block.

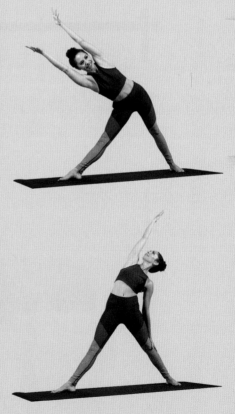

- *Extended-arm triangle*: To strengthen your abs even more, keep your torso as it is, lift your bottom hand, and reach toward the front wall, with your biceps by your ear. For more challenge, reach both arms overhead to fire up and tone your core. Hold for 5 balanced breaths or more. Bring both hands back to your hips. Root into your feet and lift using your core strength to stand up and switch sides.

- *Reverse triangle*: With both legs straight, flip your front palm and reach your right arm to the sky and your left arm down your back leg. Press down through your feet and lift your chest and top hand high as you lengthen through both side ribs.

Humble Warrior

About the Pose

Humble warrior is a warrior I variation. It adds a bind for chest and shoulder opening as well as a fold that requires fierce roots with your feet and legs as you press down and hug in, and surrender through your torso and head.

Alignment

- From warrior I on your right side, interlace your fingers at your lower back and create a bind.
- Bend your elbows deeply and hug your shoulder blades together.
- With your collarbones broad, straighten your arms, lift your chest, and gaze up as you inhale.
- On your exhale, bow your chest and head to the floor and hug your right shoulder to the inside of your right knees.
- Set your gaze to your back ankle and let your head hang heavy.

Modifications and Adaptations

You can use a strap, towel, or your shirt as a connector if your hands don't clasp in a bind. Create the general shape in a way that works for you, and remember to balance strength with ease.

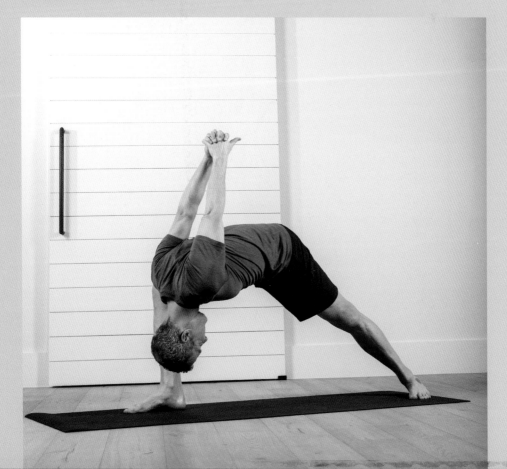

Crescent Lunge
Virabhadrasana variation

About the Pose
This full-body pose trains all of your muscles to work as one unit and helps you set your gaze and energy forward. Crescent lunge is often called high lunge.

Alignment
- With a long stance on your mat, ground down into all four corners of your front foot and stack your back heel over the ball of your back foot. Do not press your back heel toward the back of the mat. This creates a lack of integration within your body and results in loss of overall power.
- Bend your front knee to 90 degrees and align your front knee over your ankle. Straighten your back leg and firm your muscles to the bones.
- Hug your inner thighs toward your centerline, and square both hips to the front of the mat.

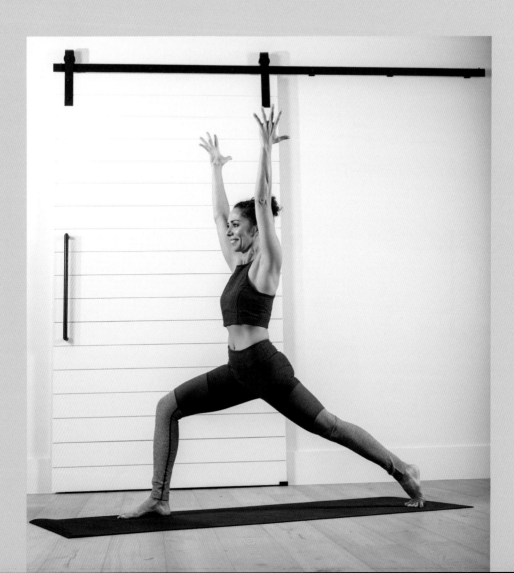

- Knit your front ribs in, slide your tailbone down, engage your core, and breathe into your middle and upper back.

- Lift your arms and chest high. Set your gaze forward at the horizon line.

Modifications and Adaptations

- *Low crescent lunge (anjaneyasana)*: Place your back knee down to your mat. Working with your back knee down can help build strength and stability with your legs, build core strength, and integrate your whole body. If you need more stability, tuck the back toes. You can place both hands on the ground for low lunge.

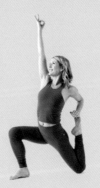

- *Low lunge with quad stretch*: Come into a low lunge with your right foot forward. Stack both hands on top of your right thigh. Hug your legs toward your centerline, engage your low belly, and shift your hips more forward. Bend your back knee and reach back with your left hand to catch your back foot. You can use a strap or towel as a connector. Continue to root down through your front foot and pull your lower abdomen in and up. Lift your sternum, widen across your collar bones, and hug your arm bones back. To come out of the pose, gently release your back foot, place both hands to the ground, and step back to downward-facing dog. Repeat on your second side.

- *Low crescent lunge with a bind*: Interlace your fingers at your lower back. Bend your elbows deeply to access your upper back and hug your shoulder blades in toward your centerline. As you inhale, straighten your arms, stretch your hands toward the ground, and lift your heart and your gaze high.

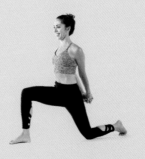

> continued

> continued

- *Lightning lunge*: In your lunge, align your chest at a 45-degree angle and squeeze your shoulder blades. Either sweep your arms back along your sides, with your palms facing the earth and your fingers spread wide, or extend your arms up, with your biceps by your ears. Create one long line of energy from your back heel through the crown of your head. Hug your outer shins in toward your center and pull your lower abdomen up and in. Your back knee can be up or down. Lightning lunge can be added into a flow on an inhale or exhale depending on your sequence.

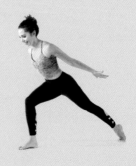

- *Fire lunge*: From a full crescent lunge, set your left knee to the mat. Untuck your back toes and press the top of your left foot down into the ground. Build your strong foundation, plug into your mat through all four corners of your right foot, and pull your heel toward the back of your mat. Activate your legs, squeeze your inner thighs, and pull into your centerline. Lift your arms and your chest high. On your inhale, lift your left knee up off the earth. Set your drishti and generate your full ujjayi breath. Continue to squeeze your inner thighs together, anchor your tailbone down, and activate your core. Feel the heat build in your legs, butt, and core as you tone and strengthen. Hold for 10 full breaths or more and switch sides.

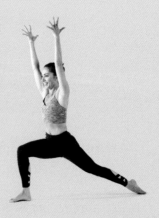

Star Pose
Utthita Tadasana

About the Pose
Star pose lengthens, opens, and energizes the whole body. This is a great transitional pose within a mandala sequence as you turn to face the opposite end of the mat.

Alignment
- Step your feet wide apart, facing the long edge of your mat, and spread your arms up and out to the sides. Align your ankles under your wrists.
- Press down into your feet and pull up through your legs and core.
- On your inhale, reach out through the fingertips, lift through the crown of your head, and expand your body out in all directions, like a five-pointed star.

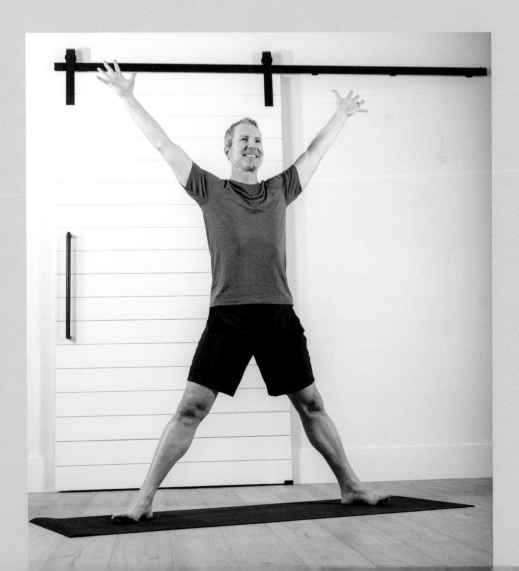

Wide-Leg Forward Fold
Prasarita Padottanasana

About the Pose

This wide-standing fold increases flexibility as it stretches and strengthens the inner legs, calf muscles, hamstrings, and muscles along the spine. It's a great stretch for runners, cyclists, and other athletes with tight hamstrings. The folding action tones the vital abdominal organs, calms the brain, and creates a deep release.

Alignment

- Take a wide stance facing the long edge of your mat, with your feet about four to five feet apart. Turn all 10 toes to face the wide edge of the mat, align your feet parallel, and straighten your legs with a slight bend in both knees.
- Catch your hips with your hands, hug your arm bones back, and on your inhale, stand tall and lift your chest.

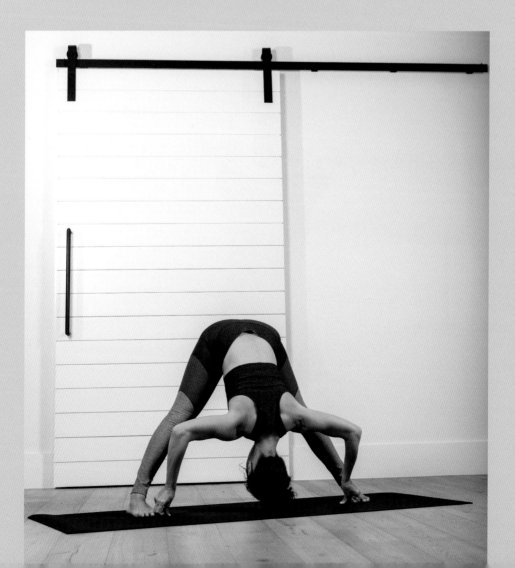

- Press down firmly through your heels, lift your kneecaps and engage your thighs, and slowly fold forward with your exhale. Shift your weight slightly forward to align your hips with your heels.
- Bring your fingers to the ground for support or use your index and middle fingers together to hold your big toes and pull your elbows wide to use your arm strength to deep your fold. Drop your head and let your neck unravel.

Modifications and Adaptations

- Use blocks underneath your head or hands to help lift the earth to you for more support. Try bending your knees slightly to lessen the intensity of the fold.
- *Wide-leg forward fold with arm variations*: Walk your fingers to line up with the arches of your feet and press up onto your fingertips. Interlace your fingers behind your back to create a bind to open and rinse your shoulders; or seal your prayer hands at your back into reverse namaste to open your shoulders and strengthen your wrists. Your fingers can be pointing up or down your back.

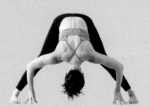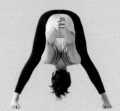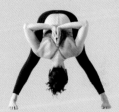

Big Toe Pose Leg Lifts

About the Pose

This variation of big toes pose elevates a forward fold into a strengthening lift. Press down into the floor and lift your core to power up your leg.

Alignment

- Step to the top of your mat in a standing forward fold, your feet hip-width apart.
- Unite your peace fingers, your index and middle fingers, and slide them between your big toes and second toes and grab hold of your big toes.
- Press down into all four corners of both feet, and inhale lift your chest into a halfway lift. Firm your leg muscles.
- Shift your weight onto your left foot and stack your left hip over your heel.
- Lift your right thigh bone into your hip and float your right foot a few inches off the earth.
- Activate your glutes and leg muscles, lift into your core, and extend your right heel up and in line with your right hip. Repeat on the other side.

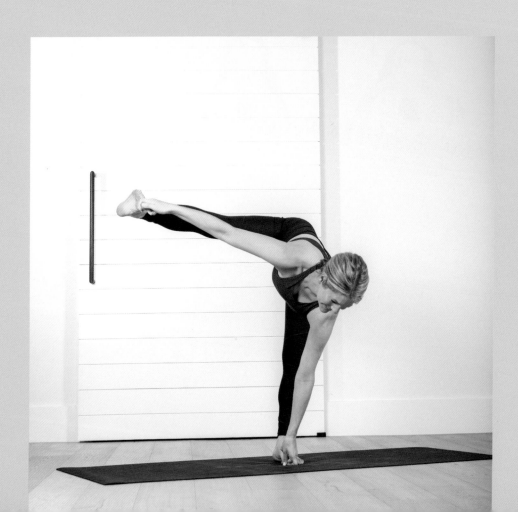

Pyramid Pose
Parsvottanasana

About the Pose
This pose translates to "intense side stretch." It tones the legs, gets deep into the hamstrings, improves balance, releases the spine, and inspires self-reflection.

Alignment
- From your warrior II or triangle legs, step your back foot up toward the top of your mat a third of the way to shorten your stance.
- Straighten both legs while keeping a slight bend in both knees.
- Bring your hands to your hips and steer both hip points forward to face the front of your mat. Squeeze your inner thighs.
- On your inhale, lift your chest high and slightly arch your back.
- On your exhale, hinge at your hips, fold forward over your front leg, and drape your belly button over your front thigh. Release your hands to the ground.
- Relax your neck and set your gaze to your back foot. Keep your eyes open as you breathe deeply.

Modifications and Adaptations
- Set your blocks on both sides of your front foot and use them as support for your hands in your fold.
- *Reverse Namaste pyramid*: Before you fold forward, spread your arms wide and unite your palms at your back in a prayer position to open your chest and shoulders and strengthen your wrists.

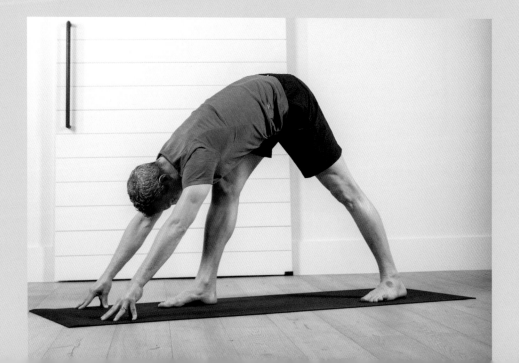

Goddess
Utkata Konasana

About the Pose
Goddess is a squat that builds heat, tones the legs, and opens the hips.

Alignment
- Come into a wide stance with your feet about one leg's distance apart. Turn your legs and toes out about 45 degrees.
- Bend your knees deeply to create a 90-degree angle and press your knees toward your pinkie toes. Pull your lower abdomen in and lengthen your tailbone down.
- Stack your shoulders over your pelvis as you reach the crown of your head toward the sky.
- Unite your palms together at your heart.

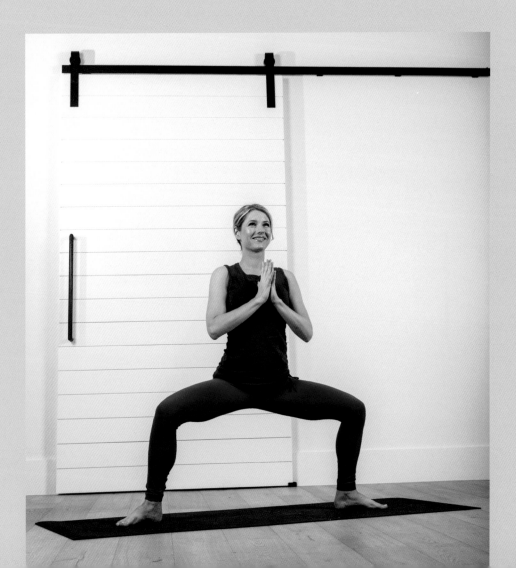

Modifications and Adaptations

- *Goddess with eagle arms*: Work arm variations into longer holds. Try eagle arms for shoulder opening.

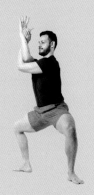

- *Goddess twist*: Press your palms into your thighs and dip one shoulder to center. Repeat on the other side. Hold for 5 to 10 breaths or add simple movements with breath.

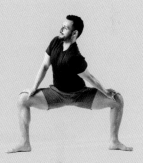

- Try adding some organic movement as you shift slightly from side-to-side or forward and back and continue to ground through all four corners of your feet. You can also use this pose as a transition in a flow on an exhale.

Big Toe Pose
Padangusthasana

The big toe pose is a standing forward fold that stretches the hamstrings and lower back.

Alignment

- With your feet hip-width apart and parallel, ground down through all four corners of your feet.

- Hinge at your hips to fold your torso over your thighs and release the crown of your head toward the ground.

- Connect your index and middle fingers together, and slide them in-between your big toes and second toes. Grab hold of your big toes. On the inhale, lift halfway and extend through your crown, lengthening your spine.

- On the exhale, hinge at your hips and fold forward. Use your arm strength to help you fold deeper by pulling your elbows out to opposite sides. Bend your knees as needed to lengthen your lower back as you rotate your inner thighs back. Tilt your hips toward the sky and stack them over the tops of your heels.

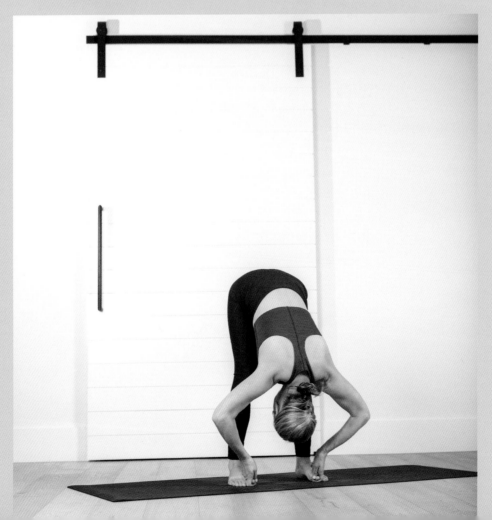

Gorilla
Padahastasana

About the Pose

Gorilla is another type of standing forward fold that lengthens and strengthens the hamstrings and lower back and puts gentle pressure on your hands to release your wrists.

Alignment

- In a standing forward fold, slide your palms under your feet with your toes facing the heel of your hands and your toes up to the creases in your wrists.

- On an inhale, come into a halfway lift.

- Stack your hips over your heels. Let your head and neck hang. Soften the muscles of your face.

- With your exhale, fold back down into a standing forward fold.

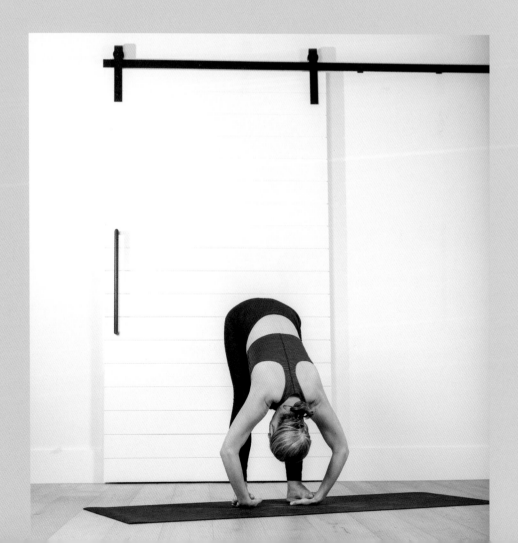

Fire Toes Pose

About the Pose

Fire toes pose will stretch and open all the muscles of your feet. You can also add some arm variations, like eagle arms or arm circles linked with breath.

Alignment

- Come into a kneeling position on your heels. Tuck your toes under and sit back on your heels.
- Hug your inner ankles together, squeeze your legs toward your centerline, and lift your hands to prayer.
- Slide your tailbone down, lift your lower abdomen, and breathe as you feel the transformative fire in your feet. Hold for five deep breaths or more.
- To come out of the pose, bring your palms to the ground, untuck your toes, and flap out your feet on your mat.

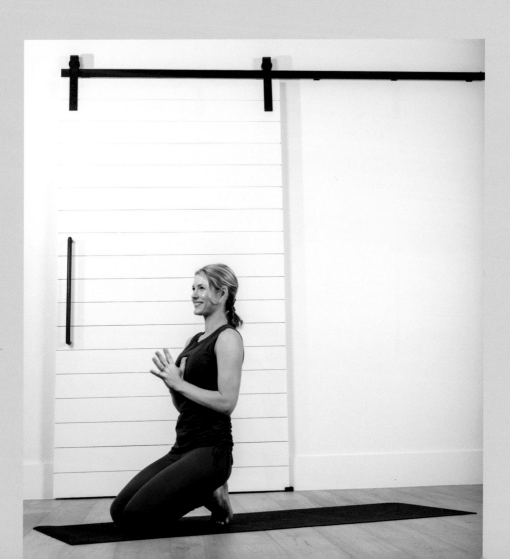

Yogi Squat
Malasana

About the Pose

This squat in most of the world is a common shape in daily life. However, for many of us who spend hours each day at a desk or driving a car, this squat can be a deep stretch for the hips, groin, and lower back.

Alignment

- Separate your feet wide enough so that both heels are on the ground as you come into a squat. This may mean lifting your hips high, and that's OK. Adapt the squat for your body.

- Press down into all four corners of your feet to create a solid foundation.

- Bring your hands to your heart center and press your triceps into your legs and your legs back into your arms. Use this connection to stabilize and lengthen your tailbone down.

- Lift your lower abdomen up and in and reach your chest high to meet your prayer hands.

Modifications and Adaptations

If squatting feels difficult, try sitting on a block for more support.

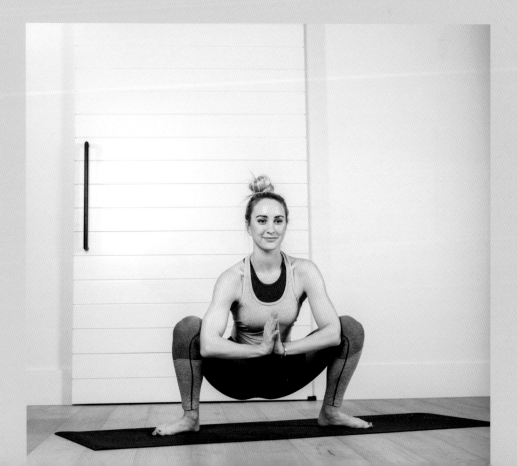

Bear Pose

About the Pose

Bear pose is a fusion between chair pose and yogi squat, and it builds serious strength and opening in the legs and hips.

Alignment

- From yoga squat, press down into the floor and lift your hips in line with your knees. Squeeze your heels in toward the center of your mat.

- Interlace your fingers, extend your arms long, squeeze your triceps into your ears, and press your palms away from your hips. Align your chest with the ground and create a line from your hips through your palms.

- Gather your power into your core, lift your belly, and expand your breath into your side ribs and back body.

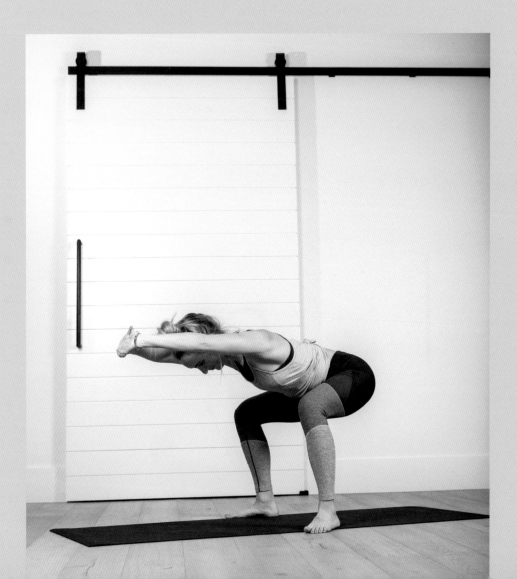

TEACHING TIP

Effective Sequencing

Sequencing a yoga class is both a science and art. With your sequences and cues, as a teacher you are directing someone else's life force energy. There is a lot of information and opinions on how to properly sequence classes, how to inform the body for peak poses, and how to follow the rules and traditions of yoga. Expert teachers and teachers in studios all over the world share a lot of incredible creativity. In power yoga, we honor the traditions as well as our own unique physical and energetic needs and goals. Don't worry about breaking the rules of yoga or doing it the way you've been taught or have always done it. Instead, learn the principles and use them to guide your experimentation. The point is that there is no one way to build into any pose and no one way to practice yoga. Every time you get on your mat, you'll gain new understanding about how to get into poses and how your body works, and so will your students. The practices in this book provide you with well-rounded sequences to build into peak poses and tips to create sequences that empower you to master poses that are calling you. As a teacher, it's essential that you study the art and science of yoga, be committed to your practice, and ultimately make sure that what you offer creates real results for your students. When you share what feels empowering and good to you, it carries energy and will make you a more powerful and authentic teacher.

Balancing Poses

Balancing poses demand your full attention and presence. These poses require a combination of effort and ease as well as strength and surrender because they teach you how to be balanced and centered through challenge and turbulence. Balancing poses help you tune out distractions and tune in to what is essential in the moment.

Establish your foundation first, then build your pose from the ground up. If you lose your balance, fall out of the pose, or get frustrated, simply begin again at your base. The pose is not the destination; the reward is what you learn within the pose and the balance you create in the process of the pose. Learn to cultivate equanimity within these poses and sequences, and you'll tap into your true power.

> When you change your focus from limitations to boundless possibilities and from doubt and fear to love and confidence, you open your world in entirely new ways.
>
> Baron Baptiste

Eagle
Garudasana

About the Pose

As you stand on one leg in this balancing bind, you'll tone your legs, open your hips and shoulders, and stretch your upper back. This pose demands your full presence as you balance with strength and ease.

Alignment

- Standing in tadasana, set your drishti to a point that doesn't move before you begin. Setting your physical gaze gives you a physical anchor for this balancing pose.
- Bend both knees and shift your weight onto your left foot.
- Lift your right leg and wrap your right thigh around your standing leg. Either slide your right foot around your left calf or touch your toes down to the outside of your standing leg.
- Repeat on the other side (shown).

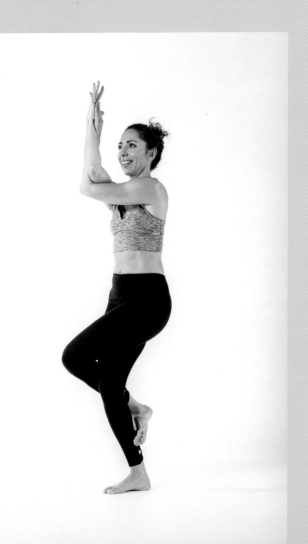

- Tilt your tailbone down toward the ground and lift the front of your pelvis up toward your belly button. Engage uddiyana bandha.
- Stack your shoulders over your hips, like you are sitting straight in a chair, and lift up through your crown.
- Wrap your right arm under your left arm and spiral your forearms. Point your fingers to the sky and unite your palms.
- Lift your elbows in line with your shoulders and stack your wrists over your elbows.

Modifications and Adaptations

- *Eagle with arm variations*: To modify, hold opposite shoulders or press your forearms together.

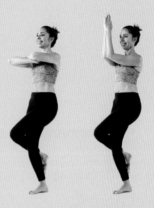

- *Nested eagle*: Crunch your elbows down to touch your knees, hug everything in, and pull your lower belly back. Shift your gaze down to the floor. This can be used as a transitional pose in a flow on an exhale.

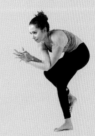

Standing Leg Raise

Utthita Hasta Padangusthasana

About the Pose

Standing leg raise tones and stretches the legs and opens the chest, and has many variations. Set your gaze to a stable point to ground your vision in this challenging balance pose.

Alignment

- Stand at the top of your mat, your hands on your hips.
- Root down through your left foot, lift your right knee up to hip level, and flex your foot.
- Either hold your right knee with your right hand, or your right big toe with your right peace fingers and extend your foot forward. Stabilize your center by pulling your belly button in and up.
- Draw your upper arms bones onto your back and broaden across your chest.
- Set your gaze straight ahead at the horizon.

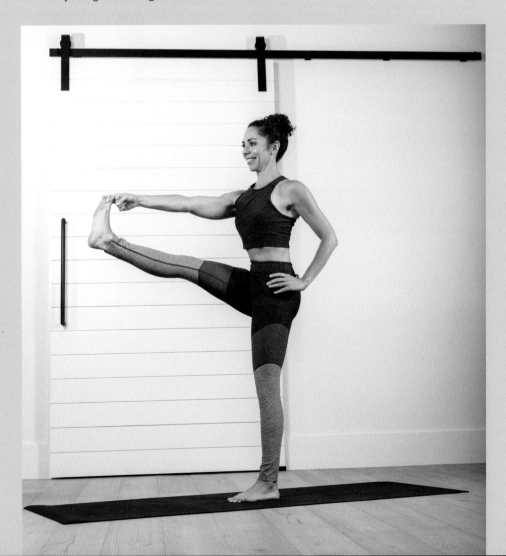

- To modify, you can always bend your knee, hold your knee, or use a strap.

- If you find yourself hunching over with your leg straight and rounding your shoulders, bend your lifted knee and pull your shoulders back. Maintain the lift of your chest and integrity of your spine rather than compromising the wholeness of your pose just to grab your foot.

- *Standing side leg raise*: Rotate your right leg out to the right side. Keep your heel away from your body as you flex your foot and firm your leg muscles. Either keep your left hand on your hip for more stability or extend your left arm. Lift through your crown as you expand out in all directions.

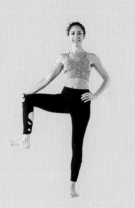

- *Standing leg raise twist*: Start in standing leg raise and face forward. Switch the grip of your hands and hold your lifted knee or foot with your opposite hand. Twist, extend the arm of your lifted leg, and reach to the wall behind you. Walk your gaze along the side wall and set your vision to your hand reaching back. Root down through your standing foot and lift up through the crown of your head. Look forward to the front wall, slowly unwind, and return to center.

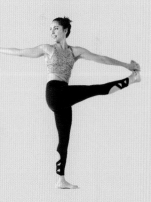

Tree Pose
Vrksasana

About the Pose

Tree pose creates balance and stillness in the body and mind, opens space within you, and invites your intention to take root. It tones the legs, strengthens the lower body, and improves overall balance. Tree pose trains you to be firm in your foundation while adapting to the changes in weather that naturally occur.

Alignment

- Standing at the top of your mat, ground down through all four corners of your right foot and lift your left foot to the inner thigh of your standing leg. As you root down, lift through the crown of your head.

- Stabilize your center by pulling your belly button up and in and slide your tailbone down.

- Unite your palms to prayer position at heart center and bring your intention back to the forefront of your mind.

- Draw your upper arm bones back and broaden across your chest.

- Repeat on the other side (shown).

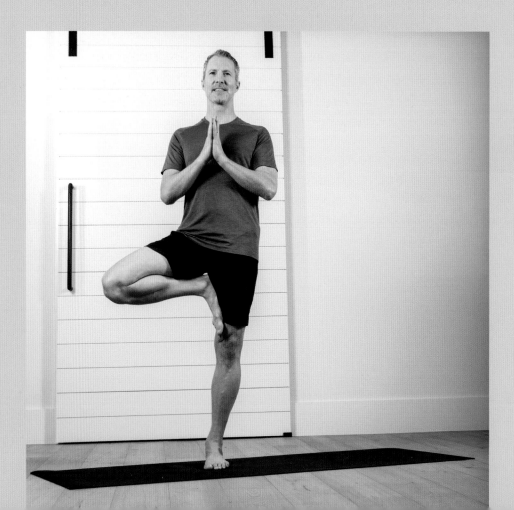

Modifications and Adaptations

- To modify, you can bring your lifted foot to your calf or even rest your toes on the ground and your heel against your standing ankle.

- Your arms are the branches of your tree. Create a shape that feels good and emphasizes the focus of your practice. You can extend your arms overhead, create a shoulder-opening bind at your back, interlace your fingers and press your palms to the sky, or move organically.

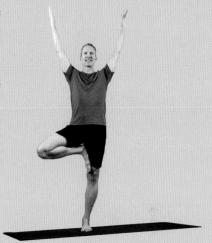

Dancer

Natarajasana

About the Pose

Dancer pose cultivates grace, focus, and power as you balance your effort with ease. This pose teaches us how to be grounded and stable while building strength, balance, and poise. As you come into the pose, set your vision to one point and remember your intention.

Alignment

- Anchor down into all four corners of your right standing foot.

- Ignite and lift your quadriceps.

- Bend your left knee and catch the arch of your left foot with your left hand. Keep your thumb facing up to ensure that your shoulder stays open. Extend your right arm to the sky.

- Tilt your tailbone down toward the ground and engage your core to stabilize at your center.

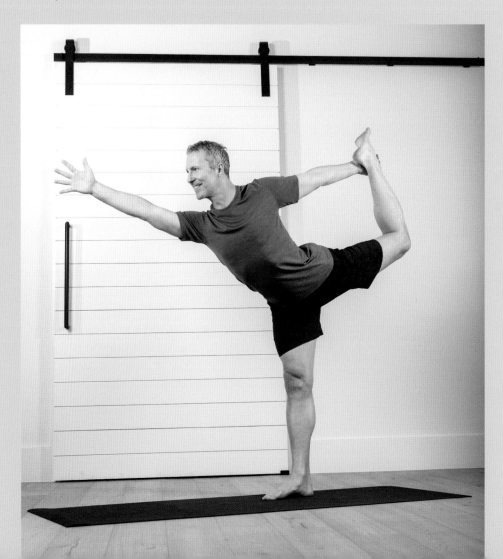

- Hug both knees toward your centerline, and with your inhale, kick your lifted shin behind you. The power of this standing backbend comes from leg strength. Lift up through your chest, top hand, and lifted foot.

- Gracefully release your lifted foot and return to standing to recenter. Transition to the other side. Hold for 5 to 10 breaths or work into a flow.

Modifications and Adaptations

Dancer with flexed foot: Flex your lifted foot and align your toes at twelve o'clock. Just like you would when standing on the ground, with press through all four corners of your lifted foot, stretch out through your toes, and power your shin to the wall behind you.

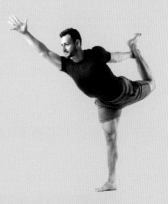

Full dancer: To add more challenge and skill, bring both hands to your lifted foot, kick up and shine your chest high.

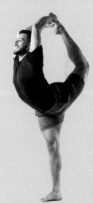

Balancing Half Moon
Ardha Chandrasana

About the Pose

Balancing half moon helps develop both stability and flexibility as you draw into your core and expand out through your legs and arms. It strengthens the ankles and legs and opens the chest. The moon carries a lot of symbolism in yoga. The sun and the moon are two opposing energies. Look to expand the lines of energy within your body as you radiate out in all directions.

Alignment

- Come into a standing forward fold to set up.
- Plant your right hand about 12 inches or more in front of your standing foot, in line with your pinkie toe, and lift onto your fingertips. Place your left hand on your left hip.
- Ground down into the four corners of your right foot, and from your core strength, lift your left leg up and in line with your hip, parallel to the floor, and flex your foot.

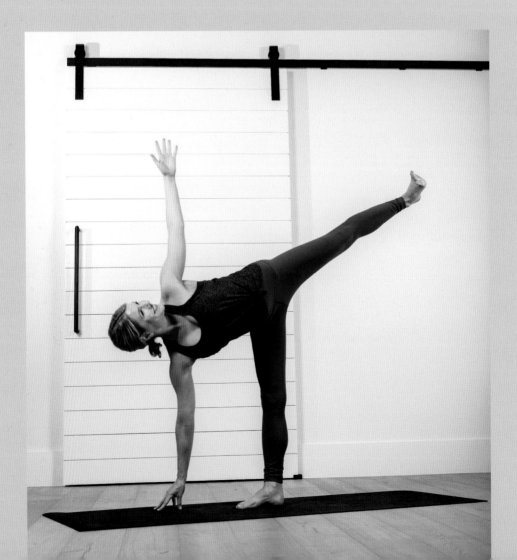

- Stack your left hip on top of your right hip and open your pelvis toward the left side wall. Activate your center by pulling your belly button toward your spine.

- You can build from here by extending your left arm to the sky, floating your top leg high, or lifting your bottom hand or both hands to heart center to cultivate even more abdominal strength. When you feel balanced and steady, slowly lift your gaze to your top hand or the sky.

Modifications and Adaptations

- If you are straining to reach the ground or your chest is facing the mat, use a block underneath your bottom hand. This will allow you to lengthen your chest forward and extend through your side.

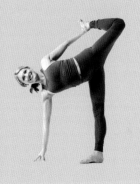

- *Sugarcane pose (ardha chandrasana chapasana)*: This variation of balancing half moon adds a front body stretch and a deep backbend. Bend your top knee and hold your foot or ankle with your top hand. Affirm the foundation of your standing foot and activate your core. Kick your foot into your top hand to create a bow and expand into new possibilities with your bind.

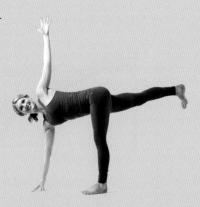

- *Revolved half moon (parivrtta ardha chandrasana)*: This variation requires you to stay grounded and balanced while adding in a deep, spacious twist. Release your top hand to the mat and square both hips to the ground, and keep your back leg lifted. With an inhale, lift your chest forward into a halfway lift, and lengthen from your back heel through the top of your head. Tone your lower abdomen to stabilize on your exhale. With an inhale, lift your other hand to the sky. Continue to lengthen on your inhales and twist on your exhales.

Warrior III
Virabhadrasana III

About the Pose

Warrior III is a pose that uses every muscle in the body to achieve stability, expansion, lightness, and balance.

Alignment

- From tadasana, use your core strength and lift one knee up toward your chest.
- With your exhale, hinge at your hips, align your torso with the earth, and kick your lifted heel to the wall behind you. Flex your lifted foot. Align both hips toward the ground.
- Reach your arms straight ahead and extend your biceps by your ears. For less intensity, you can keep your hands at heart center.
- Tuck your chin slightly toward your chest so that your neck is neutral. Set your gaze to the floor.

Modifications and Adaptations

- While still working on balance, you can keep your back toes on the mat.
- Create a bind at your lower back to emphasize leading with your chest and opening your shoulders.
- *Airplane pose*: Sweep your arms along your side, with your palms facing down and open your arms like wings. Lift your shoulder blades back and create the action of upward dog through your chest; lead with your heart.

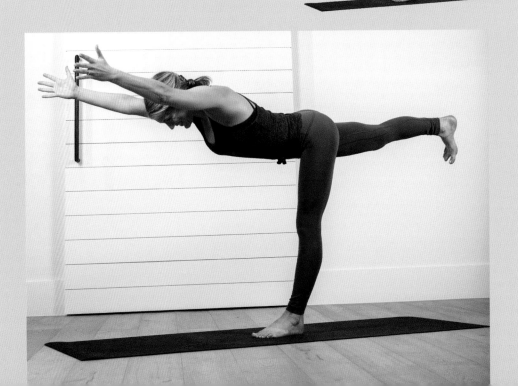

Standing Splits
Urdhva Prasarita Eka Padasana

About the Pose

Standing splits is a balancing pose, a deep hamstring stretch, and a forward fold. It strengthens the thighs and ankles and stretches the hamstrings, calves, and groin. The forward fold element helps calm the nervous system and stimulate the liver, kidneys, and vital organs. Standing splits is a great preparatory pose before a handstand within a flow.

Alignment

- Begin in a standing forward fold and ground your feet.
- Inhale, lengthen your spine into halfway lift, and press up onto your fingertips.
- Shift your weight onto your right foot. With your next inhale, lift your left leg to hip level. Roll your left inner thigh up and reach through your heel.
- With your exhale, bow your chest forward over your standing leg.
- Keep your standing leg slightly bent and lift your left leg high.
- Repeat on the other side (shown).

Modifications and Adaptations

- You can also enter standing splits from any other balancing pose or a lunge.
- Place your hands on blocks under your shoulders for more support. To intensify, bring one or both hands to your standing ankle.

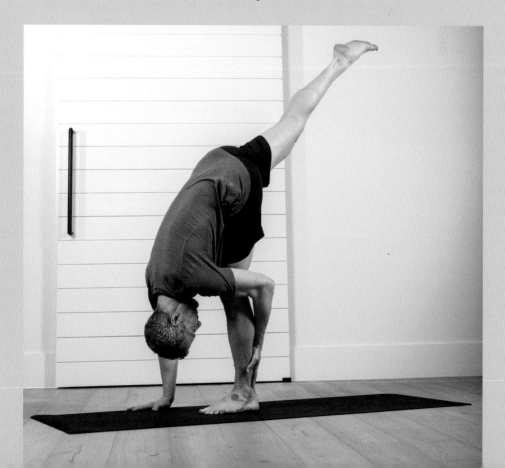

Twists

Twisting poses help cleanse the body and vital organs of toxins and excess, boost your metabolic power, and help relieve lower back pain. Twists create incredible internal massage that stimulates digestion and aids elimination. The core is the power center in the body, and core strength affects every pose. Powerful abdominal muscles help create more ease and efficiency in your movements and transitions both on and off the mat. The major energetic center at the core is ignited through twists, cultivating your inner fire and strengthening both your will and your personal power. These twisting poses and sequences will help you get deep into your core to unlock strength and lightness. To maximize the power of your twists, you must lengthen your spine before you twist to create the space for rotation.

Chair Twist

Parivrtta Utkatasana

About the Pose

Chair twist builds heat and creates flexibility and strength in the middle and lower back. It squeezes and rinses your digestive organs and kidneys. Chair twist is a powerful pose to detoxify your organs and glands, which boosts overall health and well-being.

Alignment

- Bring your feet together in the center of your mat and sit deeply into chair pose. Touch your big toes together, ground down through all four corners of your feet, and shift your weight back onto your heels.
- Lengthen your tailbone and lock your low belly.
- Unite your hands to heart center.

> continued

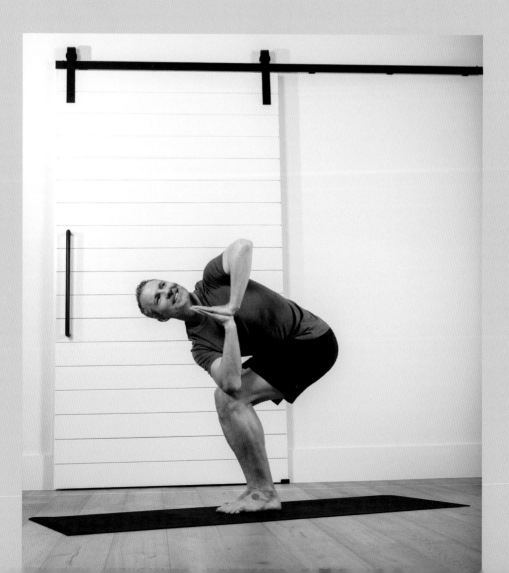

> continued

- On an inhale, lengthen your spine. On your exhale, twist and hook your left triceps over your right thigh.

- Continue to lengthen your spine on each inhale. Twist deeper with each exhale.

- Work your thumbs toward the center of your chest and lift your gaze over your top shoulder. Feel your inner heat rise as you compress and rinse your midsection.

- Repeat on the other side (shown).

Modifications and Adaptations

Open-arm chair twist: Reach your left arm forward and right arm back. Extend your hands away from one another as you open across your chest. Open-arm twists are great variations for pregnant women because these twists avoid crossing the centerline.

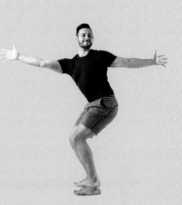

Crescent Twist
Parivrtta Parsvakonasana

About the Pose

This deep, powerful twist rinses out toxins and tension your vital organs, like your liver, kidneys, spleen, and digestive system, and infuses them with fresh energy and blood. Crescent twist improves balance; stretches the legs, spine, and chest; and increases stamina.

Alignment

- In crescent lunge, connect your hands at heart center.
- Inhale and lift your chest to meet your hands and lengthen your spine.
- On your exhale, twist. Hook your right arm over your left thigh. Press your arm into your leg to lift your torso off your thigh and lengthen your chest forward.
- Work your thumbs toward the center of your chest or spread your arms wide.
- Look up over your top shoulder.
- Ride your breath to lengthen on your inhale and twist as you exhale.
- Repeat on the other side.

> continued

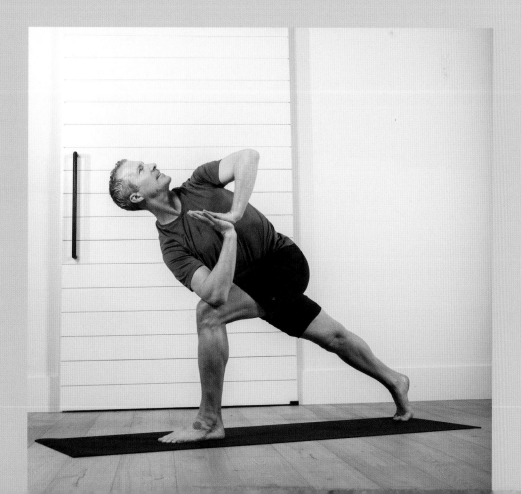

> continued

Modifications and Adaptations

- To lessen the intensity of the pose, set your back knee down to the mat.

- To create more challenge and stability, seal your back heel to the mat and work your twist with warrior I legs.

- *Open-arm crescent twist*: Reach your left arm forward and your right arm to the back of your mat. Stretch your arms away from each other and open across your chest. Maintain a long spine, with your shoulders stacked over your hips. Lengthen the sides of your torso with each inhale and twist more with each exhale.

- *Reverse open-arm crescent twist*: From open-arm twist on an inhale, turn your left palm up and extend your left arm up to the sky. Slide your right hand down the back of your left leg. Look down at your back hand, over your right shoulder, or up to your top hand. Repeat on the other side (shown).

- *Dragonfly twist*: Plant your left hand to the mat under your left shoulder, open your chest, and reach your right arm to the sky. To modify, lower your back knee to the ground. This open-arm twist is also a great variation during pregnancy.

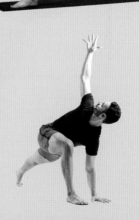

Seated Twist
Ardha Matsyendrasana

About the Pose

This seated twist stretches the shoulders, opens and energizes the spine, and stokes your digestive fire.

Alignment

- Sit on the ground and extend both legs forward.
- Bend your right knee and step your right foot over your left leg to the outside of your left thigh. Keep your right knee pointing to the ceiling.
- Slide your left foot to the outside of your right hip.
- Tent your right fingers behind your sacrum.
- With your inhale, reach your left arm high. With your exhale, hook your elbow over your right thigh.
- Hold and breathe deeply as you unwind.
- Repeat on the other side (shown).

Modifications and Adaptations

To modify, keep your bottom leg extended forward or wrap the hinge of your elbow around your bent leg and hug your torso to your thigh. For more support, you can sit on a blanket.

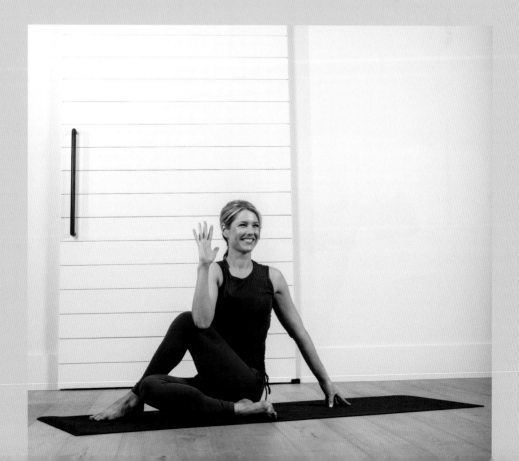

Twisting Triangle
Parivrtta Trikonasana

About the Pose

Twisting triangle is a counterpose to trikonasana. It's a twist that requires focus, balance, and skill. It stretches the legs, hips, and spine and opens the chest. The deep twist stimulates vital organs and helps relieve back pain.

Alignment

- From your triangle base, stand up, rotate both hips forward to the front of your mat, and step your back foot in a third of the way to shorten your stance.

- With your right foot forward, bring your right hand to your right hip and reach your left arm high.

- Root down into your feet and squeeze your inner thighs toward your centerline.

- With your exhale, continue to lengthen through your left side as you hinge at your hips, fold forward, and set your left hand to the mat or a block.

- Repeat on other side (shown).

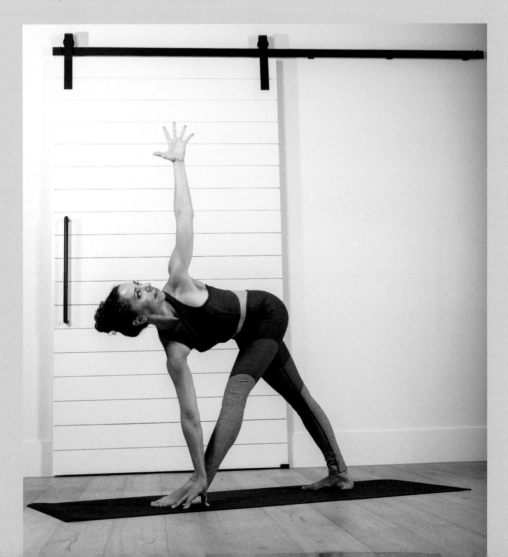

- On your next inhale, lengthen your chest forward and extend your right arm to the sky. Set your drishti to your top hand, straight to the side wall, or down at the floor.

- With each exhale, engage your core to deepen your twist.

Modifications and Adaptations

- Your bottom hand can be placed to the inside, outside, or in front of your right foot. Use a block underneath your hand to open space through your spine to empower your twist.

- It's common for newer students to have a hard time keeping the back heel grounded. If the back heel lifts, the pose can become very unstable. Try adjusting both the length and width of your stance to find the distance that works best for you and allows you to build a solid foundation with both heels firmly rooted.

Wide Down Dog Twists

About the Pose

This downward-facing dog variation adds a twist that tones your core muscles and lights your inner fire.

Alignment

- From downward-facing dog, step your feet wide, off the outer edges of your mat.
- Walk your hands halfway back to your feet and connect your thumbs at the center of your mat.
- Root down through your right palm. With your inhale, reach your left arm high and open your chest to the left side of the room.
- On your exhale, wrap your left arm under your right armpit and hold your right ankle. Pull your belly up and in on each exhale to empower your twist.
- Switch sides.

Modifications and Adaptations

Bend your knees as much as you need to in your downward-facing dog variation.

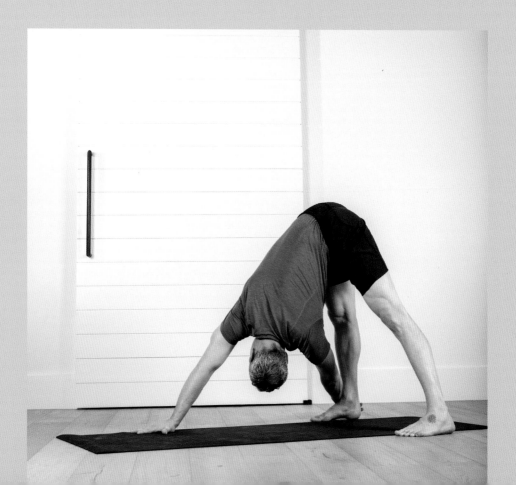

Power Sequences

After your opening sequence and sun salutations, your body is ready to go deeper. These energizing power sequences will get your heart pumping, open your whole body, strengthen your core, tone your muscles, and clear your mind. Allow your breath to lead the way as these poses help you embody your power.

I recommend using these sequences in a couple of ways. If you are just getting started with your power yoga practice, I suggest working through the sequence once on each side and holding each pose for 5 to 10 breaths, or more if you'd like. Use the sequence to get into your body. Notice the patterns and sensations you feel within each pose and how the pose changes as you hold and stay focused and steady with your breath. What you feel reveals where to put your attention. Notice where you feel coordinated and shaky, tight and open, and flexible and sturdy. The more you practice the poses and use your breath to deepen into them, the more your body will respond. Use this embodied wisdom as you progress into linking the poses in a flow of one breath per movement.

If you want to build more heat, sweat, and flow, I recommend moving through the sequence multiple times. The first time through, hold each pose for five breaths to let the pose land in your body. Use the alignment cues to detail the pose and see what unfolds and works best for you. After the sequence and individual poses are activated within your body, repeat the sequence two times or more, moving one breath per movement. Linking the poses together and repeating them with one breath per movement in a flow will increase the cardiovascular benefits of your practice, warm your body, and prepare you for what's next in your practice—backbends, peak poses, and deeper stretches.

Remember, all the poses and sequences are adaptable. If something doesn't feel right, leave it out. If you want to add or change a pose within a sequence, do it. The poses and sequence are general roadmaps for you to follow and find what feels good to you. The more you practice, the more you'll tune in to the needs of your body to restore balance and ignite the power within you.

> Do the thing, and you will have the power.
>
> Ralph Waldo Emerson

Sequencing Power

When teaching a dynamic power sequence that includes standing, balancing, and twisting poses in a flow at the pace of one breath one movement, it's helpful to guide your students through the sequence multiple times. The first time through the sequence, I recommend holding them in each pose for five breaths. Detail the alignment and actions of the pose so your students can understand how they feel within the general shape and where they sense an opportunity for growth. The second time through, lead them through one breath per movement and emphasize the breath. If the sequence is more than a few poses, I recommend breaking up the sequence. Lead them through four or five poses the first time through, then the same poses at one breath per movement, and then add poses with more breaths for exploration. Once you've led them through the full sequence a few times and have given them the whole sequence at one breath per movement, then you can set them free. This takes trust in your sequence, cues, and your students, and it creates a whole new level of empowerment for everyone involved. Let your students get deeper as they use the power poses in a dance of body and breath.

10-Minute Power Sequence

This sequence packs a lot of power in a short amount of time. It creates a full-body stretch and expansion, a shoulder and chest opening with the bind in humble warrior, and a deep balancing twist in twisting triangle. Work this sequence on the right side and then repeat on the left.

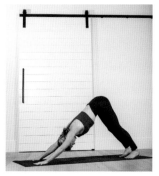

1 Downward-facing dog
(page 80)

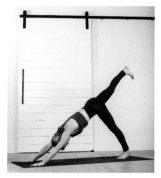

2 Down dog splits
(page 81)

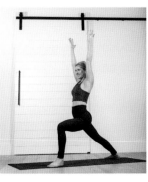

3 Warrior I
(page 91)

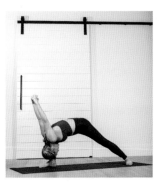

4 Humble warrior
(page 123)

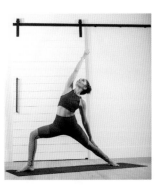

5 Reverse warrior
(page 118)

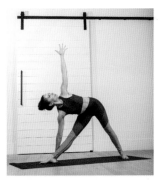

6 Triangle
(page 121)

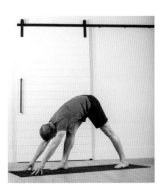

7 Pyramid
(page 131)

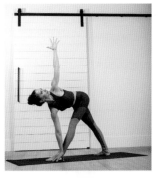

8 Twisting triangle
(page 158)

9 Vinyasa (pg. 98) to the other side

15-Minute Power Sequence

This expansive twisting sequence will create a soulful coordination of your body and breath. Move from your core in the transitions and allow your body to flow. I recommend working through the sequence the first time through to reverse warrior, then vinyasa, and repeat on the other side. The second time through, add the rest of the poses. Then repeat the whole sequence at one breath per movement.

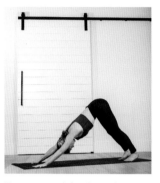

1 Downward-facing dog
(page 80)

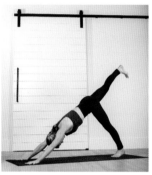

2 Down dog splits
(page 81)

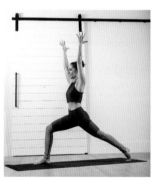

3 Crescent lunge
(page 124)

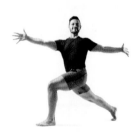

4 Open-arm crescent twist
(page 156)

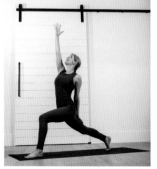

5 Reverse open-arm
crescent twist
(page 156)

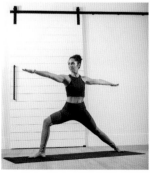

6 Warrior II
(page 117)

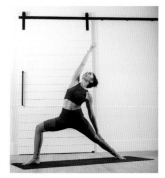

7 Reverse warrior
(page 118)

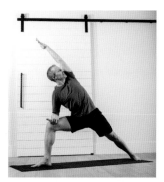

8 Extended side angle
(page 119)

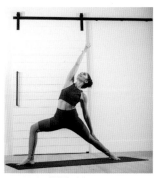

9 Reverse warrior
(page 118)

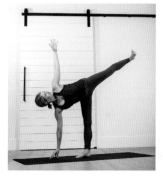

10 Balancing half moon
(page 148)

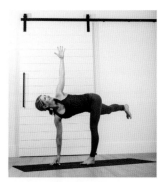

11 Revolved half moon
(page 149)

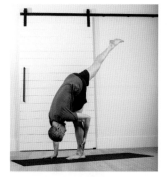

12 Standing splits
(page 151)

13 Vinyasa (pg. 98) to the other side

20-Minute Power Sequence

This sequence will build full body power and meditative focus, and you move your body with your breath. This sequence adds the element of a mandala, creating a circle on your mat as you flow. You'll turn to the back of your mat to complete the sequence on your right side and return to facing the top of your mat to complete the sequence on your left side.

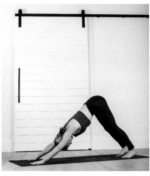

1 Downward-facing dog
(page 80)

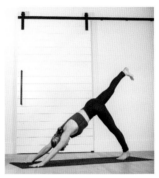

2 Down dog splits
(page 81)

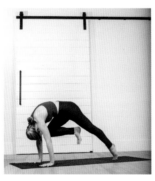

3 Down dog splits with
knee-to-nose
(page 81)

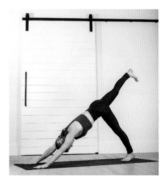

4 Down dog splits
(page 81)

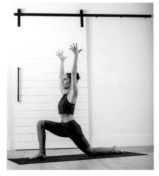

5 Low crescent lunge
(page 125)

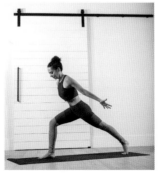

6 Lightning lunge with arms back
(page 126)

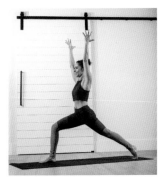

7 Crescent lunge
(page 124)

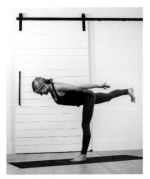

8 Airplane
(page 150)

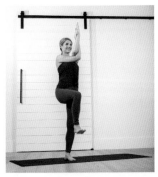

9 One-leg tadasana with left arm under in eagle arms
(page 79)

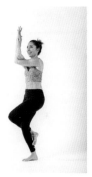

10 Eagle
(page 140)

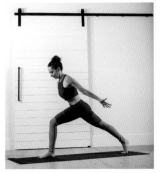

11 Lightning lunge with arms back
(page 126)

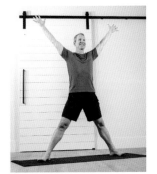

12 Star pose
(page 127)

> continued

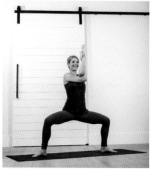

13 Goddess with right arm
under in eagle arms
(page 133)

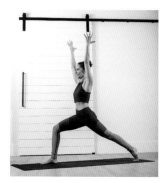

14 Crescent lunge
(page 124)

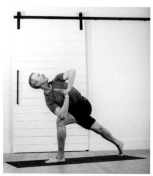

15 Crescent twist
(page 155)

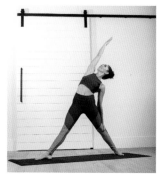

16 Reverse triangle
(page 122)

17 Vinyasa (pg. 98) to the other side

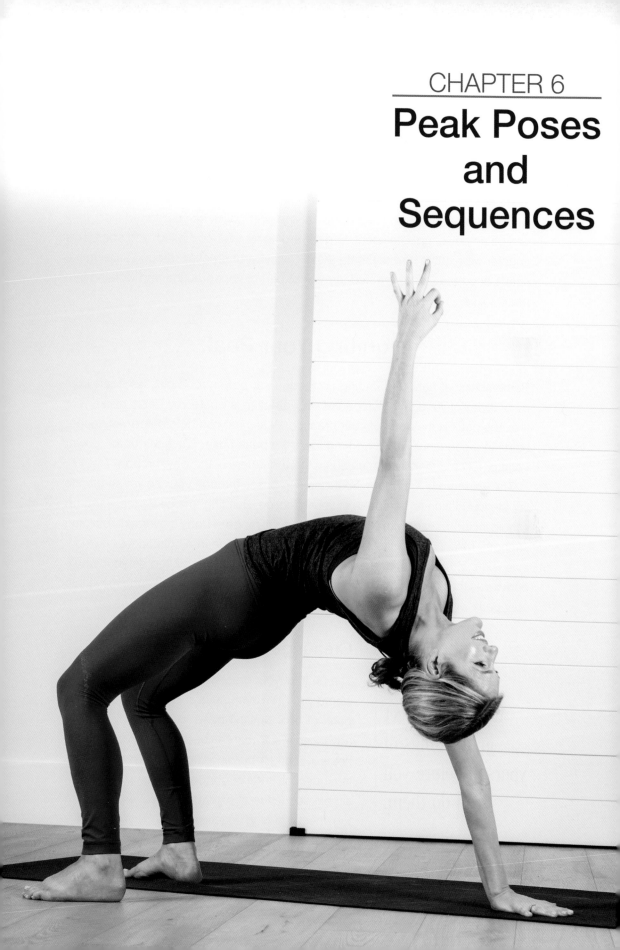

CHAPTER 6

Peak Poses and Sequences

In power yoga classes, we build to a peak pose or series of poses that require more focus, strength, flexibility, and skill than you may have in the beginning or end of class. In power yoga, the aim is to get your whole body ignited and open through your power sequence so when you get to the peak of your class, you have the freedom and flexibility to work more advanced poses. Peak poses are often the poses you see on social media or are done as party tricks. When practiced in a mindful progression with warm-ups and power poses as your foundation, they can be empowering, intelligent, and rewarding for the body, mind, and spirit. This chapter will explore how to create a peak within your practice through utilizing the space and heat you've created in the first part of your practice and working into peak poses.

Igniting Your Peak

Remember that heat and finding your edge set power yoga classes apart from other styles of yoga, and this part of your practice is where you get to utilize your fire. The peak is the apex of your practice. Peak heat can be created with longer holds in a sequence or by working toward a peak pose. The apex of the power yoga practice generally comes about three-quarters of the way through.

The warm-up is important. Your opening poses through your power sequence lay the foundation for the peak of your practice. Building to a peak, the warm-up should include a variety of poses to create a full range of body movement, building strength, balance, and flexibility and moving the spine in all directions—flexion, extension, side bends, and twists. Your breath should be ignited as your whole body feels the heat. Once you feel activated, open, and balanced, then move into your peak with more advanced asanas or challenging holds.

Creating Peak Heat

> You must expect great things of yourself before you can do them.
>
> Michael Jordan

The peak of your practice takes you to your edge, where you grow both physically and mentally. The peak of heat doesn't need to be complicated or advanced. Peak heat can be created through longer holds of strength-building standing poses, like holding crescent lunge or goddess to fire up the legs; a simple sequence of extended holds, like weaving together balancing poses to challenge your stability and focus; or targeted core work to demand more

Look for the Lights

As you begin each class, look for the most advanced student and the most inexperienced. These students are your beacons of light and will help guide you in creating a class that is both challenging and accessible for the students who have showed up for you. Teach to both, affirm them both, and help them find their edges. As you do, you'll also speak to everyone at every level within the class. Make the steps clear and give permission to stop and explore on the journey to the peak. The end pose isn't the goal; it's what your students learn in the process. Highlight the areas of opportunity and growth for every student at every level to explore what's available throughout the whole class.

of you than you think is possible. With the peak coming from heat, the goal is to stay in the poses until you feel like you can't give any more—your muscles are shaking, sweat is running down your face, and your mind is telling you to quit. Stay in the fire and with your breath and give yourself the chance to find your center during a storm. Your mind will want to give up before your body, so notice when your mind tells you that you can't take any more or that this is too much. That's the moment you can choose to stay in the pose, smooth out your breath, and access a new level of your power. In the peak, new sensations will arise as you extend the limits of your edge. Watch yourself and give a little more with each breath cycle and every practice as your strength and endurance—both of mind and body—grow.

The peak of your practice may include a variety of poses, like a few backbends and some handstand drills. Other days, you may want to work on arm strength, and your peak can be a series of planks and side planks held and linked together until you get to your edge. And some days, you may need less heat, leave out the peak entirely, and choose to move into a restorative backbend and finishing poses.

You don't have to choose a peak pose or a peak series before you begin your practice. I often get on my mat, and all I want to do is move and feel good, and I don't want to think about how to challenge myself once I build heat. Sometimes I'm not interested in choosing a higher intention or mapping out a sequence to get to a certain pose. Other times, one peak pose will drive my whole practice. Backbends, arm balances, and inversions can be worked into your practice once you establish your mind-body connection and develop heat and flow.

Your body hears everything your mind says. Pay careful attention to what you are telling yourself, especially when taking on new challenges like these peak poses. If you are telling yourself that you are going to fall before you go into crow or handstand, chances are that you will! If you repeat to yourself that something is too hard or your body won't be able to do it, then you are declaring it as so. Align your mind with the present and where you want to go. Focus on your breath and each step of the pose. Bring your attention to what you are doing and look for what is possible. Take on these challenges as opportunities for growth. There is power in aligning your thoughts with what you want to have happen, rather than what limits you. The body and mind work as one.

Working Into Peak Poses

Mastering more advanced poses isn't as simple as just doing the pose. It takes time to prepare and open the body and understand the component parts to create the whole.

When working into a peak pose, it is helpful to have a sense of where you are going before you begin so you can create a skillful sequence with purpose and power. In your warm-up and power poses, introduce actions and a variety of poses that prepare your body for the peak pose. Explore the relationship between the poses and how each pose affects what comes before and after within the sequence. Look for the patterns in shape, body part, energy, and intention. Consider what needs to be warmed up, opened, and engaged to prepare you for the apex of your practice and pick one or two key actions that will drive this home. Small details and repetitive actions help lay the foundation for your peak pose and allow you to find new power and purpose in familiar motions. Thread these movements through your practice to open specific muscles and understand the activation of the peak pose.

> May your
> choices reflect
> your hopes, not
> your fears.
>
> Nelson Mandela

Build your warm-up sequence around the actions required for your peak pose. Choose an opening pose and sequence with gentle and expansive movements that inspire your peak. For example, opening the spine with cat and cow can be helpful at the start of your practice if you're moving into wheel pose as your peak, which requires warming up all the back muscles and opening across your chest and front body.

Sun salutation variations are great opportunities to weave in physical themes that progress into your peak pose. If you are working up to backbends like wheel, you can add a side stretch within your sun salutation A's. In your sun salutation B's, you can hold your warrior poses longer to activate and use the larger muscles of the legs that are essential to wheel pose. You could also add humble warrior to continue to emphasize lengthening the side body, strengthening the legs, and opening the chest and shoulders. As you work the component parts of each pose, you'll start to turn on and fire new parts of your body and brain and create a path to work toward the peak pose.

The process of working on the prep poses and working toward the peak pose will make you stronger. Your body will create the pose that is exactly what you need in every practice, so enjoy what you can do and be patient. It's not all about the final pose. There is no need to force anything, and you don't have to "get anywhere" in your practice. It's a practice, not a posture race.

Consider these tips for working peak poses:

- *Do the pose more than once.* Repetition builds new awareness and power. Notice what feels different and what you learn each time you practice the peak pose. Spend some time "working" the pose and see what unfolds as you build alignment and practice the principles.

- *Go with your gut.* If your intuition leads you to get into a pose using a different approach, try it out. There's no one way to work a pose that will work for

TEACHING TIP

Theme to Empower

A theme is an incredible tool for teachers to underscore the actions, intention, and energy of the peak of the class. The theme can be a spiritual, philosophical, or energetic thread that you weave through the practice, much like the actions that support the peak pose. For example, if you are working up to an inversion as your peak pose, you can speak to conquering fears, the trust and vulnerability that is required when you take risks, and the rewards of doing so. Build your sequence with poses that ask your students to challenge their fears and shake things up, like practicing sun salutations with their eyes closed. Be intentional with your theme and use your words to unite the physical practice with the deeper benefits of yoga. This purposeful thread will give your students an experience that empowers them, not just in their yoga practices but also in their lives.

While this applies mostly to teachers, you may want to experiment with weaving a theme through your practice as you develop it. Ask yourself what poses support your intention for your practice. Where can you take more risk? And what poses can you add to challenge yourself and support you in feeling good?

everybody. You build new access to the pose and muscle memory in your body every time you practice.

- *Don't be afraid to fall or fail.* Falling is part of the process, and failure is essential to growth. Look for the wisdom in each fall and put it in your learning the next time you try the pose. You have to know your edges to find your center.

Peak Poses

Peak poses call for more flexibility, finesse, and focus as you reach the apex of your practice. Once you are warmed up and open, you can add more challenge with backbends, inversions, and arm balances. Remember that the power is in the process of the poses and not just in the destination. Stay open to the wisdom of the journey as you balance your efforts with ease and acceptance.

Before we begin, note that a huge part of expanding your power in this practice is knowing when to challenge your limits and when to modify, adapt, let go, and move on. No pose will look the same for everybody, and not all poses are meant for everybody. Sometimes the effort outweighs the reward. Listen to your body, your greatest teacher, to know when to leave certain poses out of your practice or adapt them. It doesn't mean you won't ever do those poses, so work with your needs and conditions now. Here are some common contraindications for the groups of poses outlined in this chapter.

> Do one thing a day that scares you.
>
> Eleanor Roosevelt

The following are contraindications for backbends:

Back injury

Carpal tunnel syndrome

Headaches

Digestive issues

Heart problems

High or low blood pressure

The following are contraindications for arm balances:

Wrist, shoulder, or neck injuries and sometimes other injuries

Carpal tunnel syndrome

Pregnancy

The following are contraindications for inversions:

Wrist, shoulder, or neck injuries and sometimes other injuries

Ocular conditions

First few days of menstruation

Pregnancy, depending on the practitioner

Backbends

There is a saying in yoga that, "you are only as young and as flexible as your spine." The spine is where the major energy centers are stored, making it the energy grid for both your body and spirit. Backbends help keep the spine limber and your energy open, empowering your health and helping you age gracefully.

Backbends release vitality along the spinal column, which ignites your energy from the inside out. Backbends help you counteract the repetitive motions of modern life—like sitting at a desk, driving in a car, and looking down at your phone. These poses create suppleness in the hips and spine while strengthening, sculpting, and emphasizing structure and integrity of your whole back. Most backbends are held for 5 to 10 breaths, and I recommend repeating each pose two times or more.

Backbends are also known as heart-opening poses. These poses require courage and vulnerability as well as faith and trust because you go backward and in a direction you don't normally go. Thus, backbends help you not only move through tension and tightness in the chest, shoulders, and upper back but also clear and open more space energetically in your heart, allowing you to create deeper connections with others and follow your desires.

Locust
Salabhasana

About the Pose

Locust is a great beginning backbend. It strengthens the torso, backs of the arms, and legs as you create length and lift through your entire body.

Alignment

- Lie on your stomach with your forehead on the mat. Extend your arms by your sides and turn your palms down to the ground.
- Press all 10 toenails into the mat to engage your legs and roll your inner thighs up to the sky.
- Reach your tailbone toward your heels and engage your lower abdomen to integrate before you lift. With an inhale, lift your chest, arms, and legs.
- Reach back through your fingers and toes and forward with your chest.
- Keep your gaze down, with your neck in line with your spine.

Modifications and Adaptations

- You can keep your feet or hands on the ground and press into the earth for support as you build strength. Work on activating your upper back and lengthening through your legs.
- *Locust with a bind*: Interlace your fingers at your lower back for a bind. Bend your elbows and hug your shoulder blades in toward your centerline. On an inhale, straighten your arms and lift your chest and legs. With your feet hip-width apart, point and spread your toes.

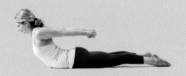

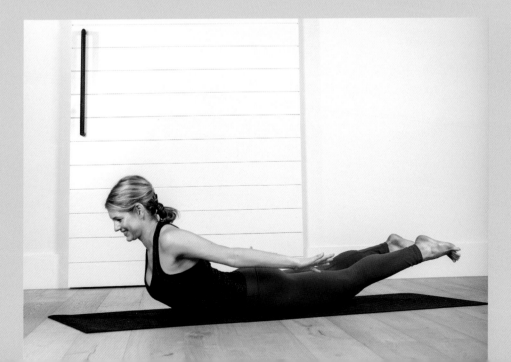

Floor Bow
Dhanurasana

About the Pose

This belly backbend is an amazing opener for the chest, shoulders, hips, and thighs. It strengthens all the back muscles, massages the digestive organs, and stimulates the kidneys and adrenals. Create the balance of effort and ease—not pushing too hard or holding back—so you can access the full benefits of your intentional breath and power that comes from cultivating balanced action from within.

Alignment

- Lie on your stomach with your forehead on the mat.
- Bend your knees and grab your outer ankles or tops of your feet, and separate your knees to hip width.
- With your inhale, kick your shins back and lift your chest with the power from your legs. Embody the energy of an archer's bow being pulled back with a strong aim.
- Press your outer shins in toward your centerline and spread your toes.
- Breathe deeply and allow your chest to open.

Modifications and Adaptations

- *Half bow*: If reaching back for both ankles feels like too much, modify into a half bow. Cross your left forearm in front of you and press down into the mat to lift your chest. Reach your right arm back to your right ankle and create a half bow and kick back. Pull both shoulder blades together as you shine your chest forward. Repeat on the other side. You can also use your strap as a connector to reach your foot and ankle.

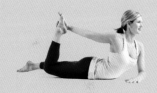

- *Floor bow with flexed feet*: Flex both of your feet and align them at twelve o'clock. Just like you would standing on the ground, press through all four corners of your feet and stretch out through your toes.

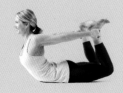

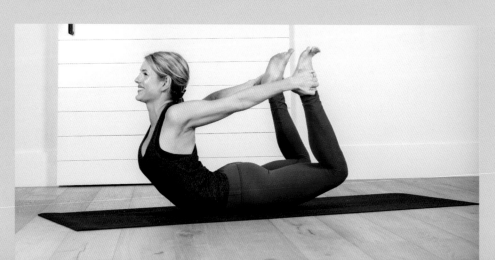

Reclined Hero Pose
Supta Virasana

About the Pose

This pose is a grounding backbend melded with a deep stretch for the hips, thighs, knees, ankles, and feet. This variation of the hero pose is best suited for later in the practice during the peak, when the body is warm and open.

Alignment

- Come into hero pose and sit on the floor between your heels. If this is too intense, let your work be sitting upright and stay seated on your props. If you feel ready to move on, start to recline.

- Lengthen your tailbone toward your knees, engage your lower abdomen, and start to lean back, and support yourself with your hands or forearms.

- Stop at any point that you feel resistance, a sign you are at your first edge. Pause there and soften into your pose.

- If you can, lean all the way back and bring your shoulders to the floor. Catch opposite elbows over your head and rest your arms on your mat.

Modifications and Adaptations

If you have any knee pain or other sharp shooting pain, recline less to reduce the intensity. In every pose, you want to be able to experience the fullness of your breath at your unique edge. This means not suffering when you feel pain and instead choosing to breathe into deep sensation.

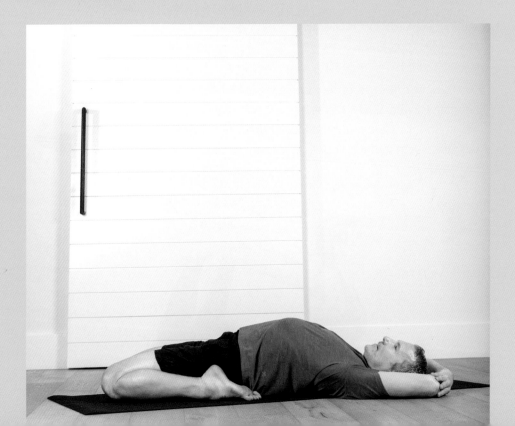

Camel

Ustrasana

About the Pose

Camel pose is a deep backbend and an energy-boosting pose. As you open across your chest and entire front body, you stimulate your nervous system and become more alert and aware. Camel pose can help relieve fatigue and anxiety and soothe headaches. Be mindful of not pushing too far or holding back in this pose so you can access the full benefits of your energy-rich breath.

Alignment

- At the top of your mat, kneel with your knees separated hip-width apart. Stand on your knees. You can flatten the tops of your feet to the mat or tuck your toes for more support.

- Connect your thumbs at your lower back, then lift your shoulders up by your ears and roll your arm bones back to open your chest.

- Press your hips forward to keep them stacked over your knees and curl your chest up and back.

- If it feels good, allow your head to drop back and open your throat.

Modifications and Adaptations

To add more challenge, reach both hands back to your heels.

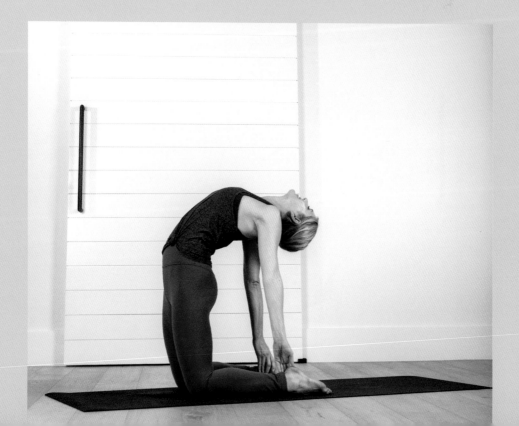

Bridge
Setu Bandha Sarvangasana

About the Pose

Bridge pose can be both strengthening and restorative. Bridge pose opens the chest, stretches the abdominal wall, and strengthens the legs. It prepares the body for full wheel pose.

Alignment

- Lie down on your back and place your feet hip-width apart, and stack your knees over your heels.
- Tilt your pelvis and lengthen your tailbone to the top of your mat.
- Ground down through all four corners of both feet and press down through your triceps.
- Inhale and lift your hips high. Wrap your inner thighs down toward the ground. Slowly lower down on an exhale.

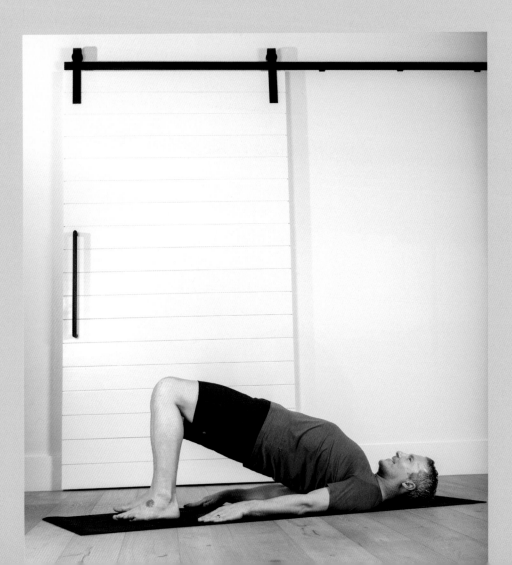

Modifications and Adaptations

- *Bridge with a bind*: Wiggle your shoulder blades in toward your centerline, clasp your hands, and interlace your fingers for a bind.

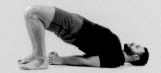

- *Bridge with one leg lift*: To intensify, root down through your left foot, bring your right knee into your chest, and extend your right heel to the sky. Hold for five more breaths with the extension, then come down and switch to the left side.

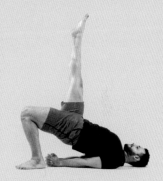

- *Supported bridge*: This passive variation of bridge opens the lower back and pelvis and can help prepare the body for more active backbends. Lie down and set up for bridge pose with your block within reach. Press down through all four corners of both feet, lift your hips up, and slide your block under your sacrum (the triangular bone at the base of your spine). It may take a few tries to find the sweet spot at the base of your spine and the height of your block that works best for you. Once you find it, settle in and allow your body to be supported by your block and your mat. Try extending your arms overhead or your legs long, if that supports you in your breath and release. Hold for 10 breaths or more to access the restorative benefits of this bridge variation. To come down, press your feet into your mat to lift your hips, slide your block to the side, and slowly lower onto your back.

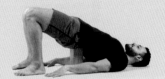

Wheel
Urdhva Dhanurasana

About the Pose

Wheel pose is a powerful and deep backbend. It requires a coordinated effort of your whole body as it strengthens the arms, legs, and spine; stretches your chest and lungs; and gives you a shot of vital energy. It expands your breath capacity as you stretch and open all the small muscles between your ribs, the intercostal muscles.

Wheel pose is both a backbend and an inversion, so you get the benefits of having your head below your heart. Because wheel pose is such a deep and dynamic backbend, make sure that you warm up and open holistically before moving into it.

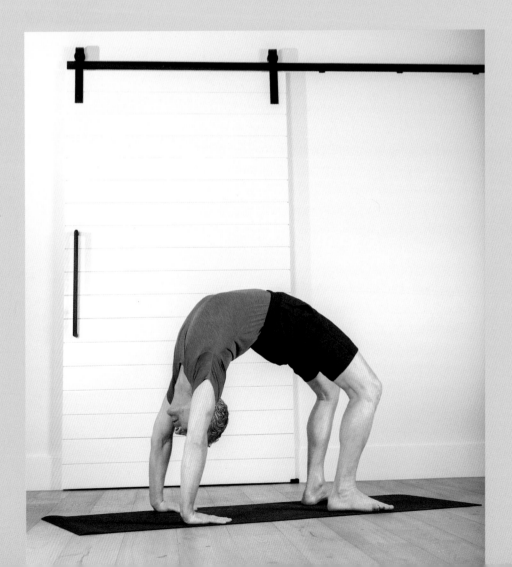

Alignment

- Lie down on your back, bend your knees, and place your feet hip-width apart, with your feet facing twelve o'clock.

- Set your palms down outside your shoulders, by your ears but wider than your shoulders, with your fingers facing back toward your body.

- Establish your solid foundation and generate your breath.

- With an inhale, press up to the crown of your head. Pause here and draw your shoulders onto your back.

- With your next inhale, press into your foundation and lift off the ground. Allow your entire front body and sides to open while you power up your back, legs, and arms.

- Spin your inner thighs down and lift your outer hip bones up.

Modifications and Adaptations

- If you feel that you are struggling to press up, try setting your hands closer to your shoulders. When your base is too long in wheel, it can feel like you are barely hanging on. There is an opportunity for more power and integration by shortening your base.

- Separate your hands a little wider than your shoulders in the setup before your press up. Draw your shoulder blades onto your back to integrate your shoulders and access more power. Sometimes going wide gives you more space for integration. With your first inhale, come to the crown of your head and emphasize this integration. Move your elbows in toward your body, hug your shoulder blades onto your back, and press up into wheel.

Flip Dog

About the Pose

Flip dog is a modern backbend variation that combines balance, core, and arm strength. It stretches the chest, shoulders, and neck as well as the hip flexors. This playful pose can help with fatigue and lift your mood and is a great backbend to add into a flow sequence.

Alignment

- Begin in downward-facing dog and root down through your knuckles to create your foundation.

- With an inhale, lift your right leg high into down dog splits.

- Bend your right knee, hug your heel toward your butt, and stack your right hip over your left hip. Flex your lifted foot and spread your toes.

- Press up to your left tiptoes.

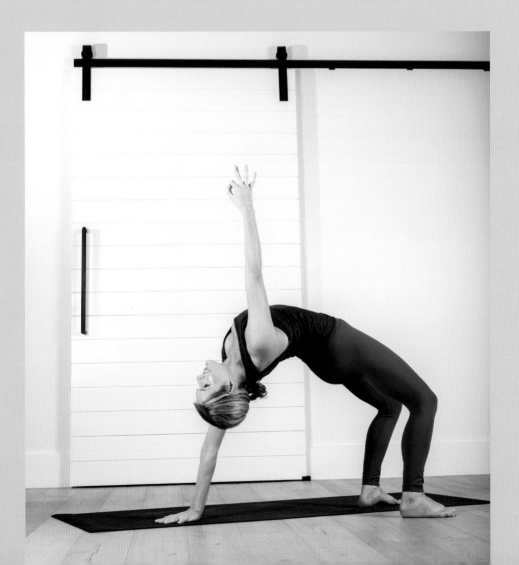

- Keep your shoulders integrated on your back, and gracefully place your right foot on the floor, with your feet aligned at hip-width facing the back of your mat. Ground down through both heels.

- Power your hips toward the sky, shine up and open.

- Squeeze the tips of your shoulders together as you expand across your chest and reach your top arm long.

- Let your head drop back, open your throat, and enjoy the expansion across your chest and front body.

- Repeat on the other side.

Modifications and Adaptations

To access a deeper opening across your upper body, bend the elbow of your lifted arm in toward your side ribs. Squeeze your shoulder blades together, lift your chest up and open, and then extend your arm with more power.

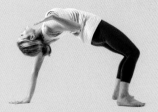

Arm Balances

Arm-balancing poses can bring a new level of challenge, confidence, and playfulness to your practice as well as develop core and upper-body strength, build bone health, sharpen your reflexes, and cultivate mental discipline. Additionally, practicing "taking flight" in arm balances can help you face fears and challenge-limiting perceptions in your life. These poses can help you move through what's blocking you and light you up in a way that you are ready for now.

Arm balances require both deep, stable roots and lightness. Developing the skill to be both grounded and buoyant empowers you to experience both qualities simultaneously in life: the balance of effort and ease and strength and flexibility. You risk a very short fall to your mat, but the wisdom that will gain in the process of trying will give you so much more.

Crow

Bakasana

About the Pose

Crow is an upper-body and core strengthener that awakens balance and lightness. Crow is a great entry pose for arm balancing.

Alignment

- From downward-facing dog, walk your feet up toward your hands.
- Press your hands down into the mat, especially your first two knuckles. Bend your elbows and create a shelf for your knees. Keep your tail high and hug your knees up high against the backs of your arms, close to your armpits.
- Set your drishti in front of your fingers, start to shift your weight onto your hands, and begin to lift your feet.
- Press the arches of your feet together and awaken your toes to ignite the power line up to your core.

> continued

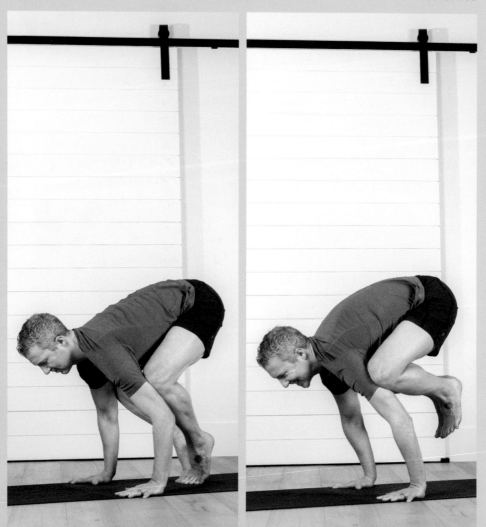

> *continued*

- Pull your heels up tightly toward your bottom. Take flight! Hold for 5 to 10 breaths.
- To come out of crow, simply bring your feet back to the ground or shoot your feet back to chaturanga and move through your vinyasa.

Modifications and Adaptations

- *Crow with a block*: To modify, step onto a yoga block, and use it as a perch for more lift. Pull your lower abdomen up toward the ceiling. You can stay here or gently work more weight onto your hands and try to lift one foot, then the other.

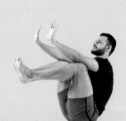

- *Seated crow*: Access the core-strengthening benefits of crow while seated. Balance on your seat in boat pose, place your fingertips on the mat behind your hips. Move your elbows back and hug your shoulder blades toward your spine line. Engage your low belly and lift your chest up and open. Keep pressing the arches of your feet together to ignite the energetic line from your feet up into your core and separate your knees wide to create crow legs. Pull the pinkie edges of your feet toward your face, press your big toe mounds away, and spread your toes. Stay in a tight boat pose variation. Lift your hands off the ground, extend your arms forward, and connect your triceps to your knees.

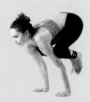

- *Crane*: In crow, straighten your arms and transition into crane pose for more of a challenge.

Side Crow
Parsva Bakasana

About the Pose
Side crow is both an arm balance and a twist. It strengthens the core, especially the obliques, and tones the arms, legs, and shoulders.

Alignment
- Start in a twisting squat, hug your knees together and balance on the balls of your feet.
- Twist your torso to the right, like in tight prayer twist.
- Plant both hands on the floor to the outside of your right leg, with your hands shoulder-width apart. Aim your fingers away from you. (This tight twist may be where you stop and work your edge as you get started.)
- Set your gaze in front of your hands and tune in to your breath.
- Bend your elbows, lift your hips slightly, and start to transfer your weight onto your hands.
- Keep your legs and feet together and use your core strength to lift your legs as one unit.
- Press down into the floor and lift into your core.
- Repeat on the other side.

Modifications and Adaptations
Step up onto a block and use it as a perch to help you deepen your twist and create lift and leverage to take flight.

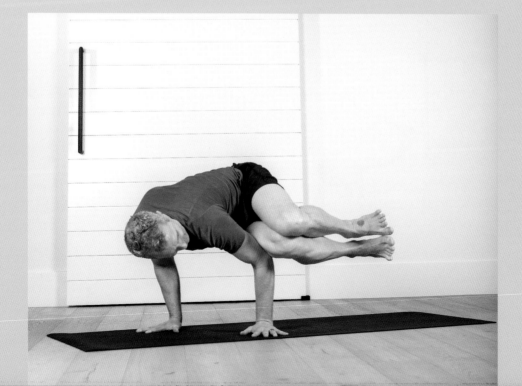

Side Plank

Vasisthasana

About the Pose

Side plank integrates the upper and lower body and uses your body weight as resistance to tone and strengthen the arms, wrists, and torso. Side plank has many variations, so build a solid foundation and create an expression that feels good to you.

Alignment

- Come into high plank pose, stack your shoulders over your wrists, and extend your heels to the back of your mat.
- Ground down through your left hand, dial both heels to the left, stack the arches of your feet, and lift your right arm to the sky.
- Look to your top hand and spread your fingers wide.
- Lengthen your tailbone toward your heels and lift the pit of your belly up and in.
- Press your hips as high as you can and open your chest.
- Flex both feet, spread your toes, and hug your leg muscles to the bones. If your feet are inactive in side plank, you are depending heavily on your arm and core strength to keep your whole body lifted. Feet, hands, and core integration are the foundation of the pose.
- Repeat on the other side.

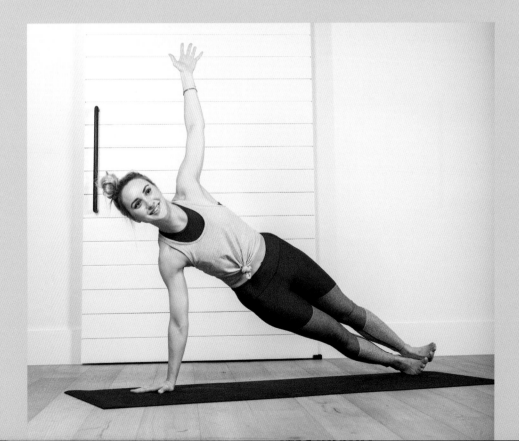

Modifications and Adaptations

- When you feel stable with your foundation, start to play with leg variations. Float your top leg up and expand in all directions or create tree pose with your top leg.

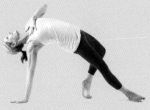

- *Wild thing*: Plant the big toe mound of your top foot behind your bottom leg and spin your chest high.

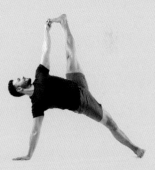

- *Full side plank (vasisthasana II)*: To intensify the pose, flex your feet, activate your legs, and raise your top leg high. Move from your core center and bend your top knee into your chest. Either hold your knee or grab your big toe or outer edge of your foot with your top hand. Extend your heel to the sky. Pull everything in and up to stabilize as you express out in all directions.

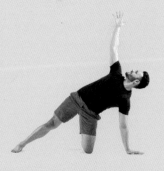

- *Plank with one knee down*: From tabletop, extend your right foot to the back of your mat, spin your heel to the ground, and stack your right hip on top of your left. Ground down through your left hand. Inhale, lift your right arm high, and expand across your heart. Gaze up past your top hand. For more support, bring your top hand to your top hip.

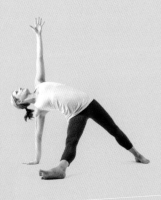

- *Fallen triangle*: From down dog splits, on an exhale, shift your weight forward onto your hands, hug in, and touch your right knee to your left tricep. Kick your right heel past your left wrist. Press down into the outer edge of your right foot and squeeze your inner thighs together. Press down through your right-hand knuckles, lift your left arm to the sky, and gaze up to your top hand. To deepen your opening and expression, you can drop your head back and reach your top arm back.

Forearm Plank

About the Pose

This pose is a modified version of a high push-up on your forearms. Forearm plank strengthens the core, stabilizes and stretches the shoulders, and tones the arms and legs. This pose is sometimes called dolphin plank.

Alignment

- From high plank, transition down to your forearms, one arm at a time. You can flatten your palms to the mat or interlace your fingers.
- Press your forearms down and soften your thoracic spine (upper and middle back) to integrate your shoulders.
- Hug into your centerline. Press your outer shins in. Firm your leg muscles to the bones.
- Extend your crown forward and reach your heels back.
- Lengthen your tailbone toward your heels and engage your lower abdomen.
- Light up your whole body, feeling everything working together as one powerful vessel.

Modifications and Adaptations

- To lessen the intensity, modify by bringing your knees to the ground.
- *Plank to forearm plank*: To build heat and strength, move up and down between your hands and forearms. From plank, place your right forearm on the mat, then walk your left forearm down into forearm plank. Plant your right palm on the ground, and then bring your left hand down to press back up to plank. Repeat this sequence 10 times, alternating which arm begins. Link with your breath. Lower to forearm plank on the inhale and press up to plank on the exhale.
- *Heel twists*: Keep both forearms sealed to your mat, and on your exhale, twist both heels to the right. Squeeze your obliques. With you inhale, bring your heels back to center. With your next exhale, twist both heels to the left. Keep twisting with breath to stoke your inner fire and build massive heat.

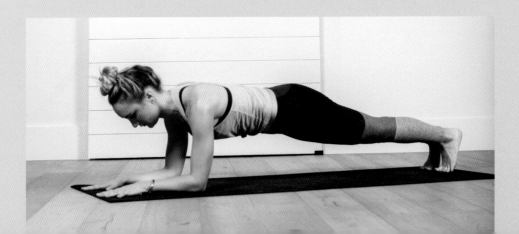

Inversions

Inversions are known for mood- and health-boosting benefits, but they're also great tools to help you break free from the seriousness of the adult world. Inversions in yoga are said to be the fountain of youth. Going upside down can infuse a sense of wonder, exploration, and play into your practice and life and can be fun and empowering.

Inversions are invigorating and rejuvenating. They promote circulation, move energy back into the vital organs, relieve physical stress on the spine, and can reduce swelling in your feet, legs, and pelvis. They positively affect all the major systems in the body—endocrine, cardiovascular, lymphatic, and nervous systems. When you put your head below your heart and reverse the flow within your body, you are literally turning your world upside down and recalibrating your biochemistry.

They can also be very calming and soothing as you create a sense balance within the poses because they require deep focus and attention. Inversions like headstand, handstand, or forearm balance can help you get out of your head and into your body. Inversions help infuse the brain with fresh energy and oxygen, which soothes and revitalizes the nervous system. As you release the muscles in your neck, you open the pathway to bring more oxygen-rich blood into the brain. As you breathe deeply in the inversion, you infuse even more energy (prana) into each breath, and more energy and blood are directed to the brain to re-energize your thinking. If you feel like you are stuck in your head or lost in your thoughts, try shaking things up and do an inversion. Flip your energy upside down and see what clarity emerges from resetting your system physically.

The more you stack your spine and joints, the easier it will be to find and create balance while inverting. You must work to establish a firm foundation—through your hands, forearms, or head—and extend upward through the feet, as if you were standing on the ceiling. Root down to grow high.

When I first started my yoga practice, inversions were difficult for me. I hadn't played on my hands in years, and I was still working through some trauma and injury from a fall when I was a college cheerleader. Once I started getting back into my body with my yoga practice, I started to crave this challenge, and I began practicing handstands with the support of a wall. I built my inversion practice outside of the studio first, and the space next to

> "We are very afraid of being powerless. But we have the power to look deeply at our fears, and then fear cannot control us."
>
> Thich Nhat Hahn

Is it safe to do inversions during your period? I get this question a lot. If you are no longer menstruating or this doesn't apply to you, feel free to skip this section. In some yoga styles and traditions, it is not advised to do inversions while menstruating. From a yogic perspective, this has to do with not wanting to reverse or interrupt the natural downward flow of energy, known as apana, during your cycle.

However, every woman is different, and no one period is the same. I suggest following the same wisdom as the rest of your practice. Do what feels best to you and adapt your practice to meet your needs. I usually don't feel like practicing at all the first few days of my cycle, and if I do practice, it's much slower and more restorative. Toward the end of my cycle, my energy shifts, and I usually feel a lot of connection to my core and like to go upside down. Listen to your body and create your practice in a way that works and feels good for you.

my desk became my handstand spot. During conference calls at work, I would press the mute button, kick my feet up against the wall, and go upside down. I felt the benefits from my inversions—I felt refreshed, renewed, and inspired after long calls, when before I would feel drained and depleted. And eventually, I was able to start kicking up to handstand in my practice in the middle of the yoga room.

Going upside down can be super fun but is not required. You can skip inversions completely or take a more restorative variation. Practice patience with yourself as you build strength and face your fears. Yoga is a journey, not a destination.

Headstand
Sirsasana A

About the Pose

Headstand is known as the king of asanas. Standing on your head with optimal alignment strengthens the whole body and refreshes the mind. Sirsasana, or traditional headstand, helps relieve fatigue and stress as you flush your whole body and brain with oxygen-rich blood and new energy. It tones the abdomen and helps improve digestion

Headstand is considered a more advanced pose, so is best suited for students with some experience in their practices. A solid base is necessary to build this pose. Once you have a strong and consistent practice, then gradually begin working the steps of headstand into your practice as a peak pose. There is no need to rush anything in yoga, and this is especially true for poses on the head and neck.

Alignment

- Kneel and bring your forearms to the floor. Connect your opposite hand to your opposite triceps to establish proper distance between your elbows.

> continued

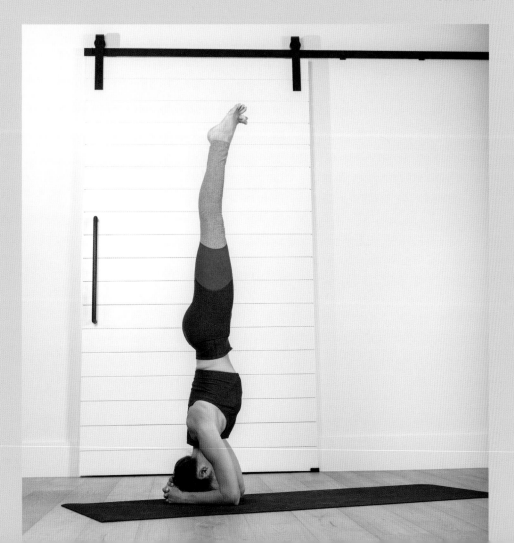

> continued

- Interlace your fingers, including your thumbs, and press the base of your palms together. It is essential to establish the proper distance of your arms to create an equilateral triangle at the base before you go up into headstand. Most of your weight should be supported by your arms.

- Connect the crown of your head to the ground with the back of your skull pressed against the basket you've made with your hands. Gaze at your knees and make sure your eyes are parallel to the mat.

- Straighten your legs and come into a modified downward-facing dog.

- Walk your feet forward toward your arms until you stack your hips over your shoulders.

- Pause and tap into the still point within your core.

- Dive into your breath and generate your flow. (This may be a great place to stop and build awareness while being upside down as you are building your headstand practice.)

- Tuck your knees into your chest and hug your heels toward your glutes.

- Press down through your arms. When you are ready, straighten your knees and bring your whole body into a vertical line.

- Create the energy of tadasana upside down. Hold for 10 to 20 breaths.

- Slowly come down, reversing your steps, or hinge at your hips and pike down. Take child's pose to reset.

Modifications and Adaptations

Once you feel stable in your headstand, play with leg variations. Trying bending both knees for pinwheel legs or eagle legs or a wide straddle.

Tripod Headstand

Sirsasana B

About the Pose

Tripod headstand delivers similar benefits as traditional headstand. It also opens the gates for many more advanced transitions and arm balances.

Alignment

- Come into table top and place the top of your head on the ground in front of your hands to make an equilateral triangle with your head and hands, and bend your arms to 90 degrees. You should be able to see your fingernails. If you can't, your base is too narrow, and you should move your hands back toward your knees.

- Tuck your toes, lift your hips, and come into a down dog variation.

- Move your feet toward the top of your mat until your hips are stacked over your shoulders. Pause here, tune in to your breath, and balance the weight between your hands and head. (This may be where you stop and explore your edge.)

> continued

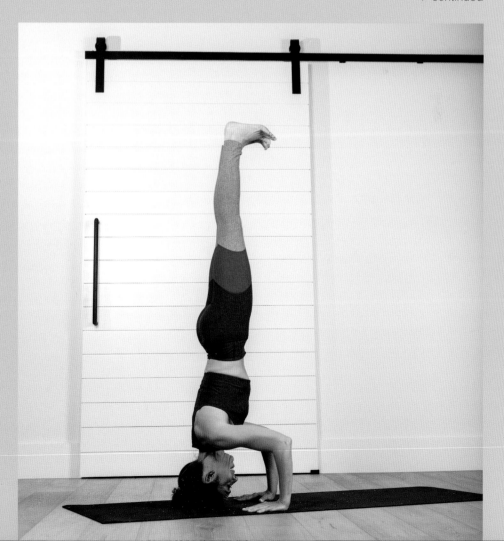

> *continued*

- Walk your knees to the backs of your arms by your armpits as if your arms were shelves. In this compact tripod, squeeze your heels to your bottom and gather your power into your center. (This is a great shape to pause and build strength.)

- Hug your legs together, keep your knees bent, and lift your knees up over your hips, with your heels still hugging into your bottom.

- Extend your feet to the sky.

- To exit, reverse the steps. Then take a few breaths in child's pose.

Modifications and Adaptations

If you feel there is a lot of pressure on your head, try putting a folded blanket under it. You can also practice both versions of headstand close to a wall for support.

Dolphin
Ardha Pincha Mayurasana

About the Pose

Dolphin pose is preparatory pose for forearm balance and has many benefits on its own. It's a deep stretch for the shoulders and upper back and strengthens the core, arms, and legs.

Alignment

- From plank pose, lower to your forearms. Walk your feet toward the top of your mat to create a short downward-facing dog on your forearms.
- Press your forearms firmly into the mat.
- Lift your gaze to between your hands.

Modifications and Adaptations

If your back starts to round, bend your knees to help create length through your entire spine.

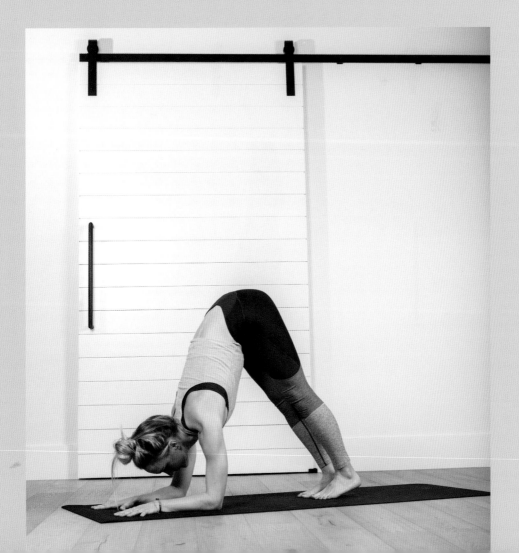

Forearm Balance

Pincha Mayurasana

About the Pose

Forearm balance strengthens and stretches the arms, neck, and upper back. It's helpful to use a wall for support as you build into this pose.

Alignment

- Come into a short downward-facing dog on your forearms, about a foot from a wall. This is known as dolphin pose.

- Set your gaze between your hands. Slowly start to walk your feet up toward the top of your mat until your hips stack over your shoulders.

- Lift your right leg up into a down dog splits variation. (If you've reached your edge, pause here, hold the pose, and breathe.)

- Exhale and hop your feet up. If you are close to a wall, rest your right heel on the wall and lift your left leg to meet your right.

- Press the arches of your feet together to unite your legs. Spread your toes.

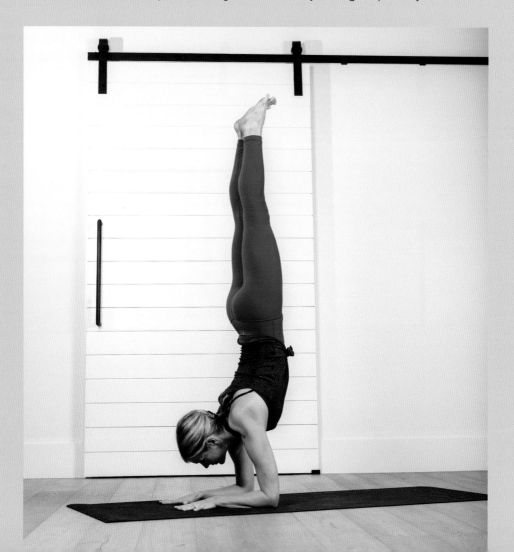

- Press down through your forearms and lift up through your heels.
- When you feel stable, slowly work one heel off the wall, then the other.
- Come down one leg at a time and switch sides.

Modifications and Adaptations

If you feel your elbows sliding away from each other as you are going up, try using a strap around your triceps to help maintain the width of your base. You can also place a block between your hands and use the L shape of your thumbs and index fingers to hug the block and pull into your centerline.

Handstand

Adho Mukha Vrksasana

About the Pose

Handstands can be fun and empowering and can give you a break from overthinking. Handstand is mountain pose, but you're on your hands. As you begin and build your handstand practice, I suggest using a wall for support. Set your base about a foot away from the wall and make sure nothing is hanging that will be in your way.

Alignment

- Walk your feet halfway up your mat and come into a short downward-facing dog.
- Lift your gaze between your hands, shift your shoulders over your wrists, and lift your right leg high.
- Bend your standing leg slightly, exhale all your air to access the strength in your core, and hop your feet up.
- You can keep your heels on a wall or try to catch some air out in the open.
- Switch sides when you feel ready. Have fun!

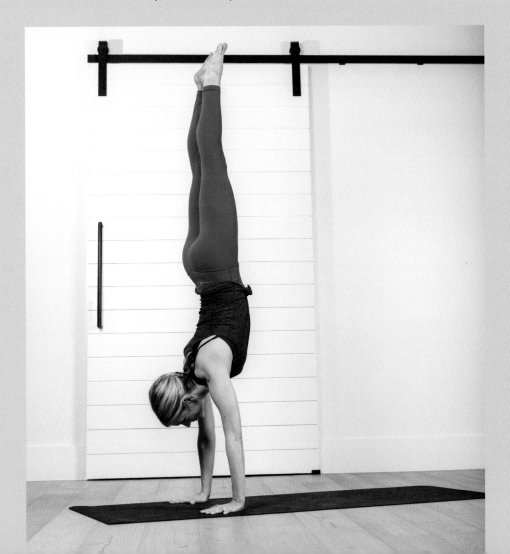

Modifications and Adaptations

- *L-shaped handstand*: Come into a short downward facing dog with your heels against a wall. Plant your hands to make roots. Bring one foot up to hip level, then lift the other foot to create an L shape, setting your feet against a wall (not pictured). Stack your hips over your shoulders and wrists. Keep your arms straight and strong as you lift your hips up to the sky. To intensify, keep your legs together, and on your exhale hop with your legs piked in to handstand, as shown.

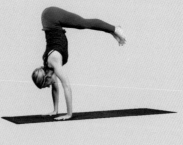

- *Handstand hops*: In your short downward-facing dog, set your drishti between your hands, stack your shoulders over your wrists, and lift your right leg. Bend your standing leg slightly, exhale your air, and hop up. Repeat a few times and then switch sides. You can also bend your standing leg into a stag to help find you balance on your hands.

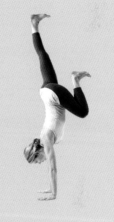

- *Handstand switch kicks*: Switch kicks build on your handstand hops. On your right side, as you exhale and hop up, switch kick your legs through handstand to land with your right foot down and left leg high. With your left leg up, hop up and land on your right leg. Keep moving for 10 rounds or more as you switch your legs, generating heat and core strength. Maybe catch some air in handstand along the way.

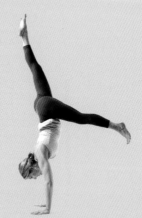

Leapfrog Hops

About the Pose

Leapfrog hops are a fun way to build the strength and skill to go upside down. Maintain a waterlike quality through your pelvis as you hop and have fun! Leapfrog hops can also be added to your sun salutations as you shoot back to chaturanga.

Alignment

- Walk halfway up your mat and come into a short downward-facing dog.
- Step your feet together to connect your arches, lift your heels, and separate your knees wide to create crow legs.
- Keep this connection at your feet to ignite the energetic line from your feet up into your core. This plugs you into your core power as you hop up and creates total body integration.
- Lift your seat high and look forward, past your fingers.
- With your exhale, hop your hips up over your shoulders.
- As soon as you come down, hop back up for 10 rounds.

Modifications and Adaptations

To build strength and confidence, you can practice these close to a wall.

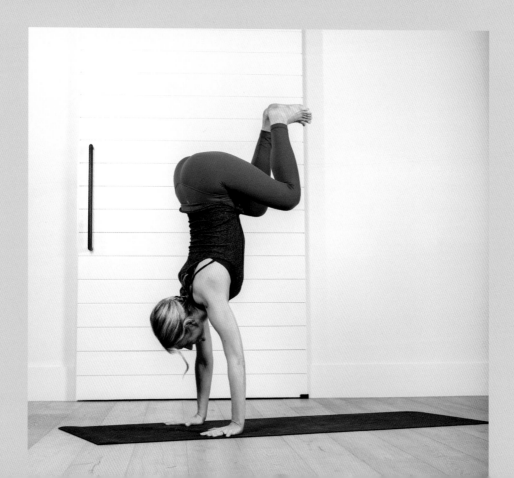

Shoulderstand
Salamba Sarvangasana

About the Pose

Shoulderstand is considered one of the most essential yoga poses. It is a reju-venating inversion that promotes circulation and helps improve immunity. It has a calming effect because it stimulates the parasympathetic nervous system, creating harmony in the body and mind. It's important to build your shoulderstand practice gradually and safely because your body weight is supported by your shoulders, neck, and head.

Alignment

- Lie on your back with your arms by your sides.
- On your exhale, press down with your arms, curl your knees into your chest, rock up onto your shoulders, and lift your hips. Wiggle your shoulder blades

> continued

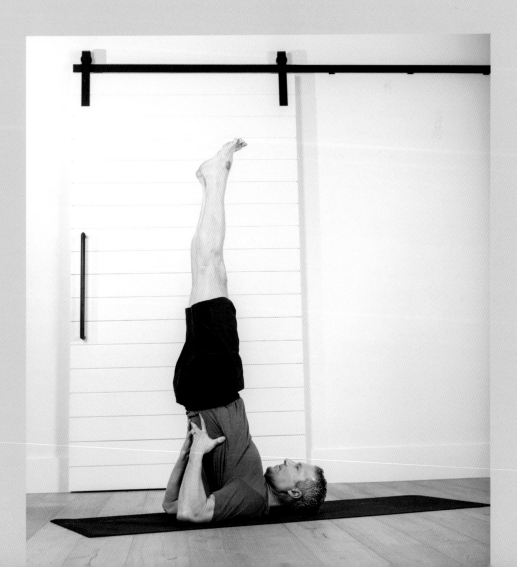

> continued

closer together and set your hand on the middle of your back to help support your hips.

- When you feel ready, extend one or both legs up to the sky.

- When both legs are lifted, hug your legs together. Flex your feet, lift through your heels, and flair your toes open.

- Set your drishti straight up and keep your neck stable and still to protect it. Make sure you lift through your heels to avoid putting too much strain on your neck.

- To come out of the pose, align your arms along the sides of your mat and make a runway for your spine. Either move through plow pose or bend your knees into your chest. Engage your core and slowly lower down to the mat, one vertebra at a time. Hold here for a few breaths and notice the impact of inversion.

Modifications and Adaptations

- If you have any neck or back problems, or feel strained in this pose, I suggest leaving this pose out of your practice for now. Legs-up-the-wall pose is a great alternative to shoulderstand.

- For more support, place a folded blanket under your shoulders. Avoid putting any props under your neck.

- *Half shoulderstand*: This is a less intense variation of shoulderstand, but you still reap the same benefits. Lower your legs to a 45-degree angle and create the shape between shoulderstand and plow pose.

Legs-Up-the-Wall Pose

Viparita Karani

About the Pose

This pose is a passive and supported inversion that allows the blood from your legs to flow back into your midsection. I recommend performing legs-up-the-wall anytime you need to restore and reset your energy. This pose is great for relieving lower back pain.

Alignment

- Scoot one hip next to a wall, lie down on your back, and lift your legs up the wall. You can also place a block or blanket under your sacrum and lift your heels to the sky.
- Let the weight of your legs set your thigh bones back and expand your lower back.
- Keep your legs active but easy and allow the energy and blood to flow from your legs to your vital organs.
- Extend your arms to your sides and allow your body to restore and rejuvenate. Turn your palms up to the sky as a symbol that you are open and ready to receive. Hold for 10 to 20 breaths or more.

Modifications and Adaptations

You don't need a wall to do this pose. Simply lie on your back and lift your legs into the air to access the same restorative benefits. You can add a block underneath your sacrum, as shown.

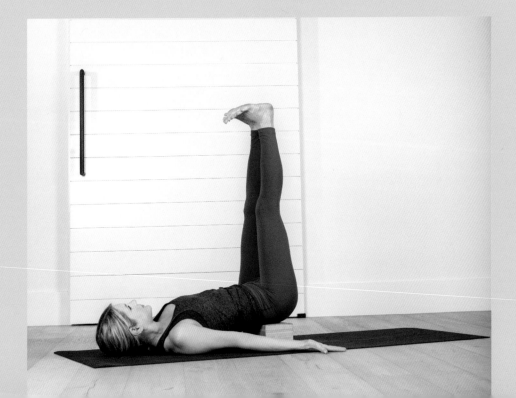

Plow Pose

Halasana

About the Pose

Plow pose is a deep back opener that stretches the shoulders and spine. It stimulates the vital organs of the abdomen and the thyroid, and can help with back pain and headaches. Plow pose often follows shoulderstand.

Alignment

- If you are transitioning into plow from shoulderstand, keep your legs straight as you slowly lower your toes to the ground. Otherwise, lie on your back with your arms along your sides.

- With your exhale, press down with your arms, roll up onto your shoulders with your hips over your shoulders, and lift your legs up and over.

- Draw your shoulder blades closer together and either place your hands on your midback for stability or interlace your fingers for a bind. Press your triceps into the mat.

- If your toes touch the ground behind you, flex your feet, firm your legs, and lift the backs of your knees skyward.

- Set your drishti straight up to the ceiling and lift your chin slightly. Do not move your head or neck while you are in the pose.

- To come out of the pose, lengthen your arms along the sides of your mat. Engage your core and slowly lower down to the mat one vertebra at a time.

Modifications and Adaptations

- If you feel any strain in your neck or upper back, hold off on plow pose for now and instead do legs-up-the-wall pose.

- *Ear pressure pose (karnapidasana)*: From plow pose, bend your knees to the outside of your ears. Keep your arms extended, or place your hands on your heels or behind your knees.

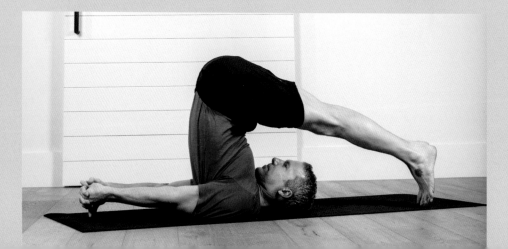

Fish Pose

Matsyasana

About the Pose

Fish pose is a powerful counterpose that releases the muscles in the back and opens the throat, chest, and entire front of the torso. Fish pose stimulates and opens the throat and heart areas, which are the centers for self-expression and communication. Fish pose is often practiced after shoulderstand and plow as a counterpose.

Alignment

- Lie on your back with your legs extended out in front of you and expand through your toes.
- Press your forearms into the mat at shoulder-width apart and slide your hands under your sit bones with your palms on the mat.
- Draw your shoulder blades toward your centerline and expand across your chest and collarbones.
- Pull your chin into your chest; then let your head drop back. Touch your crown to the floor.
- Open your throat and breathe deeply.

Modifications and Adaptations

Full-extension fish: To deepen the pose, bring your arms together above you, unite your palms, and reach your fingertips to where the front wall meets the ceiling. From your core, press your legs together and lift your feet off the earth. Spread your toes.

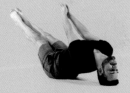

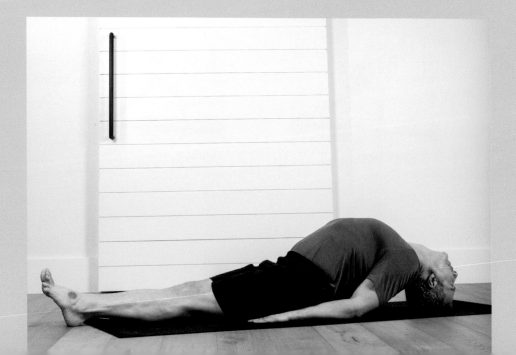

Peak Sequences

Peak sequences constitute the crescendo of your practice because you build up to this series that requires more opening, skill, focus, and heat. Before you begin these sequences or work into a peak pose, I recommend a solid warm-up with an opening sequence, a few rounds of sun salutation A and sun salutation B, and a power sequence that includes standing poses, balancing, and twists to holistically prepare and open the body. For each peak sequence in this chapter, I've included suggestions for prep poses from previous chapters to weave in the building blocks for the peak poses.

This is the peak of your practice, and it is meant to be challenging and imperfect. Allow yourself the freedom to explore bending backward and going upside down and look for the wisdom and the fun in falling down and trying again. This is how we learn and grow. As you welcome the unsteady parts of your yoga practice patience and grace, you can start to meet life as it comes, both the highs and the lows, and feel the freedom and ease that emerge from your yoga practice.

After you've hit your peak, make sure you take time to cool down, restore, and take a final rest. We'll get into the details about the finishing poses of your practice in the next chapter.

Backbend Peak Sequence: Wheel

Prep Poses

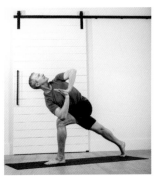

1 Crescent twist
(page 155)

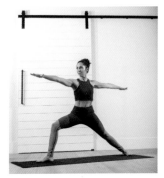

2 Warrior II
(page 117)

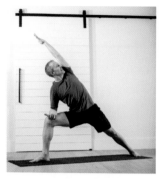

3 Extended side angle
(page 119)

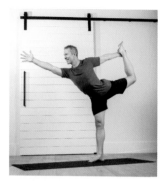

4 Dancer
(page 146)

Peak Sequence

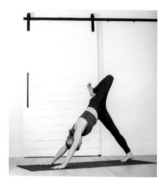

1 Down dog splits with bent knee
(page 81)

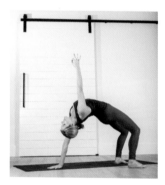

2 Flip dog
(page 184)

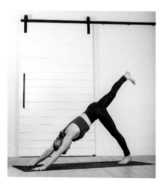

3 Down dog splits
(page 81)

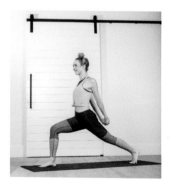

4 Crescent lunge with a bind
(page 125)

> continued

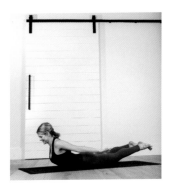

5 Locust
(page 176)

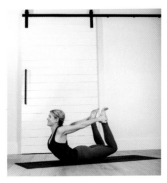

6 Floor bow
(page 177)

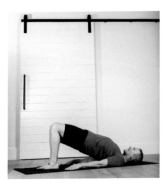

7 Bridge
(page 180)

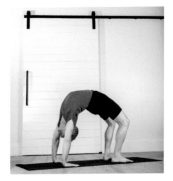

8 Wheel
(page 182)

Arm Balance Peak Sequence: Crow and Leapfrogs

Prep Poses

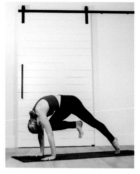

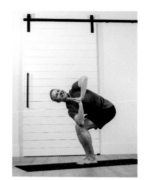

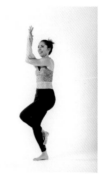

1 Down dogs splits
with plank curl
(page 81)

2 Chair twist
(page 153)

3 Eagle
(page 140)

Peak Sequence

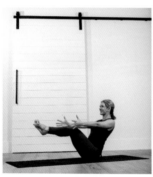

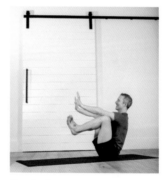

1 Boat
(page 248)

2 Seated crow
(page 188)

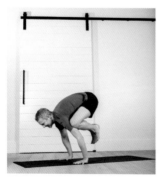

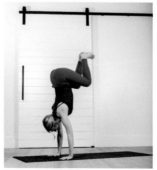

3 Crow
(page 187)

4 Leapfrog hops
(page 204)

Inversions Peak Sequence: Handstand

Prep Poses

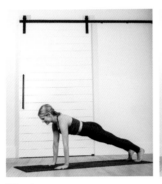
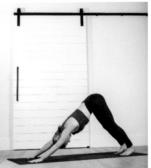

1 Plank waves
(page 251)

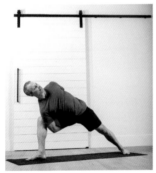

2 Extended side angle
  with a bind
(page 120)

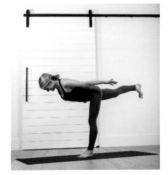

3 Airplane
(page 150)

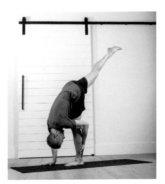

4 Standing splits
(page 151)

Peak Sequence

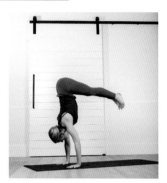

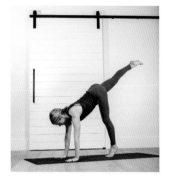

1 L-shaped handstand
(page 203)

Note that this step is done
against a wall, with the feet
on the wall (not pictured).

2 Handstand hops
(prep shown)
(page 203)

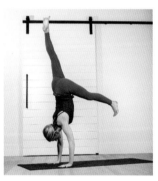

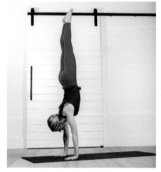

3 Handstand switch kicks
(page 203)

4 Handstand
(page 202)

CHAPTER 7

Cool-Down Poses and Sequences

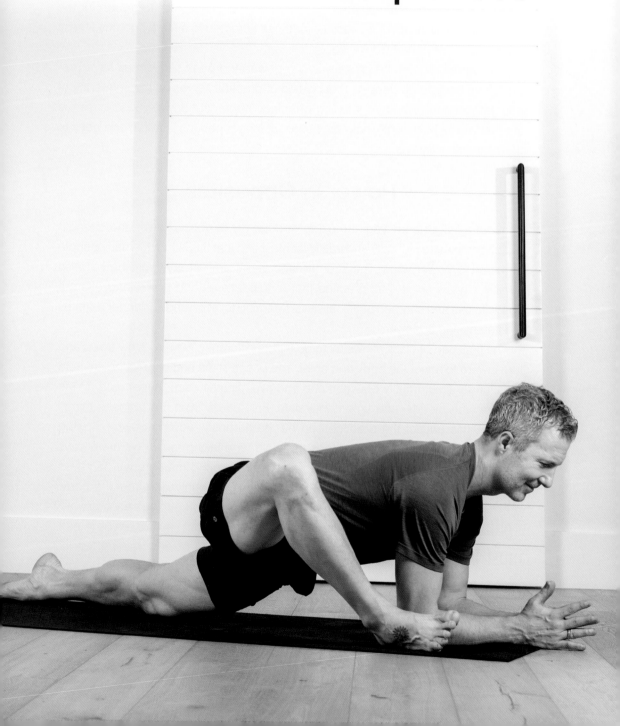

We warm up and work up to peak poses and heat, and we must cool the body down at the end of practice to neutralize the effects of more strenuous postures. Cool-down poses and practices create a holistic journey through the body at the end of powerful sequences and emphasize stretching, accepting, and letting go. Additionally, some days you'll want—or need—a cooler and more calming practice and can use these elements independently.

In this chapter, we'll move into finishing poses on the floor and focus on hips, forward folds, and final rest. This recovery and rest is essential to growth for the body, mind, and the spirit, especially for those attracted to a more rigorous fitness routine and fast-paced way of life.

The warm-ups and the intensity of the power and peak sequences have prepared the body to go deeper. This portion of practice serves as the sequence of counterposes to your strengthening practice. In the cool-down, you will use the fire that you've built within, hold the poses for longer periods, stretch, and get into the connective tissues.

Power in Opposites

I am not a flexy, bendy yogi. I have to work on my flexibility. Power and strength poses come more naturally and easily for me. I find that this is true for many people attracted to power yoga. The strength and sweat are not only enticing but also familiar. This is an athletic practice that requires focus and power and offers a space to use and sharpen physical skills. Learning to let go and surrender requires a different kind of power.

The final part of class allows us to do things differently. Now we slow down and turn inward to honor the body and spirit. The poses at the end of practice are held for a longer time, ideally between one and five minutes each, depending on the posture, your needs, and time constraints. For "doers" who like to make things happen, this part of the practice can be the hardest—slowing down, allowing things to unfold, and taking rest. If we are always moving fast and powering through, we can miss the subtle shifts in communication from the body. You can learn much by doing things another way. This is especially valuable if you are a type A personality. At the end of the power practice, we let go of strengthening and lengthening, and shift into sensation and surrender.

> It is not enough to climb the tree; we must be able to get down, too.
>
> T.K.V. Desikachar

Hip openers and folds allow a deeper conversation with the body through sensation and breath and stimulate the subtle (energetic) body. In these introspective poses, let your body be your guide to greater sensitivity, deeper awareness, and inner wisdom. These poses require the opposite of doing: allowing. Allow yourself to feel what's buried, allow the practice to unfold within in you, and feel what you feel without doing anything about it. You have to be willing to let the pose happen. If you are holding back or resisting the pose, it can feel like a struggle. Just breathe, be in the experience, and watch how the pose opens for you and how you open in the pose. As you listen to your body, it will respond by helping you go deeper into poses and give you more freedom and peace physically, mentally, and emotionally.

These poses should be both well-structured and restorative. Build the shape and alignment to support you in creating release. Start by activating the muscles opposite the area that you want to stretch. For example, in forward folds, you lift your quadriceps to stretch the hamstrings. You can certainly stay in active stretches for shorter periods with the muscles engaged, and this is great to do when you have a limited time for your practice. However, I've found the greatest power in my own practice and in what I share with my students in holding enough space at the end of a fiery practice for longer, deep holds and surrender. Once you've settled into your breath and the structure of the pose, then progress into a practice of release. This shift into more yin energy—longer holds and passive poses—creates an embodied understanding of the union of opposites within the body.

All things in life have an opposite: yin and yang, hot and cold, light and dark, masculine and feminine, sun and moon, stillness and movement, tension and release. *Yoga* means "union" or "to bring things together," so it's important to explore the opposites within your practice to create a whole and complete experience. As we expand and strengthen physically in power yoga, we must close and soften to cultivate balance in the body and mind. Both energies are necessary to create a power and wholeness.

Yin yoga is a slower, meditative method based on the meridians of traditional Chinese medicine. It targets the deep connective tissues within the body, the fascia. Fascia supports and surrounds all the major systems, muscles, joints, and organs of the body. It is a protective and connective layer that contains nerves and affects the energy of the body and mind. While this web of connective tissues has long been appreciated in Eastern traditions, it has recently started to be considered in the West.

Connective tissues are tough and fibrous and don't respond to quick and rhythmic movements the way muscles do. The texture of fascia is often compared to that of taffy. If you pull slowly on two ends of a piece of taffy, you can eventually stretch and mold it. However, if you try to quickly pull it apart, the taffy will snap and break. The same goes for tissues deep within the body. They work much more slowly, so you have to access them in a different way, and in yoga, this happens through heat and time. At the end of a heat-producing power class, there is a unique opportunity to relax the muscles and get into the connective tissues around the muscles, bones, and joints. Because power yoga is a modern interpretation of yoga, I've found incredible power and results in adapting the practice of yin yoga and combining it to complete an active power practice. Yin and yang together creates a holistic and complete practice.

The intention is to relax and release in these poses, but that doesn't mean they will be easy or pain-free. It's quite the opposite. As you get into the deep tissues of the body, these poses and longer holds can be some of the most confronting, painful, and therapeutic parts of the power practice.

This inward focus, both physically and energetically, is the fifth limb of the eight-limbed path, pratyahara, in practice. When you turn off external stimulation, you can get quiet and look within. As you slow down and turn inward, simply watch the fluctuations of the mind. Notice what comes up for you. What repetitive thoughts show up: boredom, anxiety, frustration, fear? Are old memories or emotions stirred up? Rather than being caught up in the flurry of chatter from your mind, simply meet it all with breath and accept what is and what is showing up.

Every experience we have is energetic and leaves an imprint on the body. How deep of an impression depends on the experience, circumstances, and person, and sometimes old memories and emotions, when not fully processed or released, can be stored by the body. Each time you get into deep sensation, you are in the process of active transformation. When you feel the sensations within the pose, use your breath as a tool for clearing. With each breath and level of release, you can start to unwind and unravel years of tension and layers of old energy. As you breathe and surrender, you'll melt away old holding patterns, habits, and limits of body, mind, and spirit. Use the poses to get into the body, and use the breath to unravel the knots within.

> The breath is the intelligence of the body.
>
> T.K.V. Desikachar

When you feel it and confront it—energy, emotion, tension, tightness—you can choose to either keep the energy within you or move it out and let it go. Your exhale is the pathway for purification. With a calm determination, meet sensation with your steady, equanimous breath and know that this, too, shall pass. Temporary discomfort is part of the process of letting go. It's part of a bigger journey to more freedom in your body and mind.

On your inhales, fill the space between your ribs. Use the inhale to expand from the inside out and make space to move into. The exhale is your key to release, let go, and move old energy out of your body that you no longer need. With each exhale, stretch a little further and allow yourself to melt into the pose. Muscular release in the body encourages mental release from everything else in your life.

It takes time to settle into poses, so be patient with your body and areas where you feel tension. I suggest holding these poses for a minimum of 10 breaths and up to 5 minutes. I've had some of my most transformative moments on my yoga mat during this part of the practice, when I've let go of the doing and the trying, and I've allowed my body and mind to be one with my breath.

Notice when your mind wanders off or you get lost in a storyline. It's the nature of the mind to want to pull you out of your experiences. Every time your mind tries to take the lead, return to your breath and your body. Remember that yoga is a system of bringing the mind back to the present moment. It's not about control; it's about letting go and being fully in the present moment.

Off the mat, when we resist or avoid feeling uncomfortable, hold back from the unpleasant or intense experiences, or overthink things, we often miss out on the richness of life. Life requires us to adapt and evolve, and transformation is a process that can be messy and emotional. And so much of life is out of our control! Yoga teaches us to accept and embrace things as they are, rather than resisting or trying to change things. The more you allow yourself to be with things as they are, the more you build your power. It takes energy to micromanage situations, relationships, or yoga poses until it all meets your liking. The more you allow yourself to feel the intensity of a situation, face it fully, and breathe deeply and purposefully in the center of a storm, the more you'll be able to do this in stressful situations in life. You are building muscle memory—and emotional strength—within yoga poses.

Yoga gives us the opportunity to find peace in the way things already are, and that includes our bodies. When we give up the idea that something needs to change, we can move past perceived limitations. And when we love ourselves as whole and complete, we realize the goal of yoga.

> Learn to let go.
> That is the key to
> happiness.
>
> Buddha

Hips

To clear out tension and tightness in the body often means working through the hips. Hips are like the emotional storage closets for our bodies, where we hold old tension, stress, and memories. In hip-opening poses, we're "unpacking" the body by focusing on areas we may avoid in our day-to-day activities. Once you work through the clutter and density in the hips, freedom and clarity of body and mind become available. The cleansing power comes through surrender and moving energy with breath through the dense fibers of the hip muscles.

The intention of these poses is to open and release, so know that you will hit inner resistance along the way. Tension in the body is stuck energy. Send your breath to the parts of your body that are calling out for more attention and use the tools you've cultivated throughout your entire practice as you shift from dynamic movement into powerful sensation.

If you feel fidgety or anxious within hip poses, know that is energy being stirred up from the pose. Choose to meet this energy with your calm, steady breath. As you breathe through any discomfort, it starts to melt away, and you step into new space for growth and release. Once you settle in, choose to stay still and make simple adjustments only as needed. Just feel what you feel, be with the sensation, and simply breathe into the depth of your hip stretch. Meet each moment in these deep, longer holds with acceptance for things to be exactly as they are and watch what unfolds in your body as you allow your mind to quiet.

Frog
Mandukasana

About the Pose

Frog pose stretches and releases the deep tissues of the inner thighs, groin, and hips. It can be very intense because it targets tissues that aren't often accessed through daily activity or in other poses. Because of this, frog pose can unlock energy and emotions held deep within the hip fibers. Release is available, but only if you are willing, so choose to trust your breath and allow yourself to unwind and relax in this pose.

Alignment

- Come to all fours and then down to your forearms.

- Widen your knees as far apart as you can, with your thighs perpendicular to your torso and bend your knees to 90 degrees. Make right angles from your hips to your knees to your ankles. Flex your feet.

- Tune in to your steady breath, then create the arm position that supports you at your edge. You can stay propped up on your forearms, stack your hands to create a pillow to rest your head, bring your chest down to the floor and extend your arms out wide, or slide a block under your chest for some support. Create the shape that is comfortable enough to stay in the fullness of your breath for a few minutes.

Modifications and Adaptations

There shouldn't be any pain in your knees. If there is pain, try adding more support under your knees by rolling in the edgings of your mat or placing blankets under your knees. If you still feel knee pain or if you are working with a knee injury, try the pose against the wall and on your back.

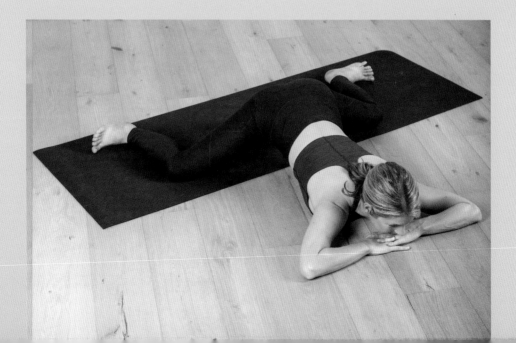

Half Pigeon
Eka Pada Rajakapotasana

About the Pose

Half pigeon is an extremely effective stretch for the piriformis muscle in the front leg of the pose and for psoas with the back leg. These muscles are often tight in runners and athletes and hold tension from sitting and other daily movements.

Alignment

- From downward-facing dog, step your right foot toward your left wrist, place your right knee toward your right hand, and lower down to the mat. Flex your front foot. In this external rotation, the more parallel your shin is to the top of the mat, the deeper the pose. You can slide your right heel closer to you to adapt to your needs.

- Extend your back leg straight behind you. Square both hips forward and walk your hands to the outside of your hips and press down through your fingertips to lift and open your chest for a few breaths.

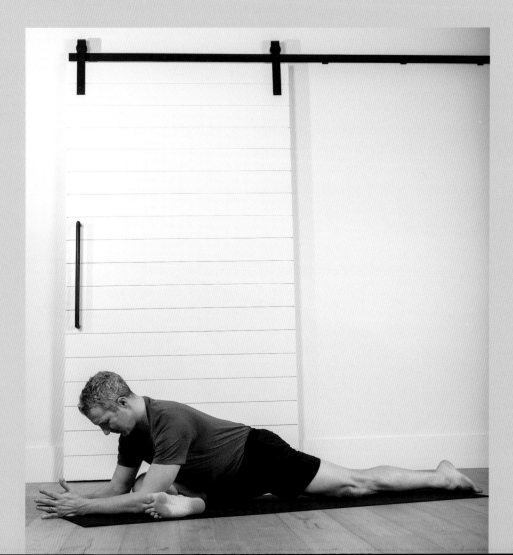

- Draw your inner thighs toward your centerline and pull your power up and in.
- On an exhale, crawl your hands forward and fold into half pigeon. Rest your forehead on the earth or prop yourself up on your forearms.
- Channel your breath down into your hips and lower back. Lengthen your whole body with each inhale and melt toward the floor with each exhale.
- To finish, walk your hands back and sit upright and repeat on the other side.

Modifications and Adaptations

- If the hip of your front leg lifts off the ground, slide a block under your hip for support.

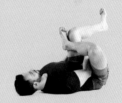

- *Reclining half pigeon*: This is a great variation if you are working with a knee injury or feel any pain in your knees. Lie down on your back with your knees bent. Cross your right ankle over your left thigh. Thread your right arm through the hole between your legs and hold either your left shin or your hamstring with both hands. Flex both feet and pull your legs toward your body. You can use your right elbow to press your right leg away from your body to help you get deeper into the muscles of your seat. Send your breath down into your hips, butt, and lower back. Repeat on the other side. This pose can be great in your opening sequence for a more hip-centered practice.

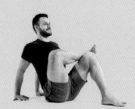

- *Seated half pigeon*: Begin while seated and place your hand behind your hips. Lean onto your fingertips. Sit up tall, and roll your shoulders back to open across your chest. Bend your knees and plant your feet on the ground. Cross your right ankle over your left thigh and flex your foot. You can walk your left foot closer to your or further away to find the degree of stretch that feels best for you. Press your top knee away from your chest.

Double Pigeon
Agnistambhasana

About the Pose

Double pigeon, or fire log pose, is an intense stretch for the hips, especially for the piriformis muscle. This pose can take some time to work into, so give yourself the space to allow this pose to unfold with your breath.

Alignment

- In a seated position, stack your right shin on top of your left shin, with both legs parallel to the top of the mat.

- Flex your feet and keep the heat and stability through your legs.

- Press your hands down by your hips and scoot your hips back a few inches to help tilt your pelvis forward.

- Lift your heart high as you inhale and broaden your chest.

- Hinge at the hips and ride your exhalation down to fold forward. Rest your forearms on the ground or on a block. Release your head and neck.

- Slowly bring yourself back up, reverse your legs, and repeat on the other side (shown).

Modifications and Adaptations

- If you feel you are at your edge, you can work the pose sitting upright. Try going up onto your fingertips with your hands behind your hips to help lift and lengthen your upper body.

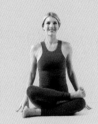

- If you want to intensify, slide your top ankle bone to the outside of your bottom knee. Fold forward and release your head and neck. Turn your palms up to the sky as you completely surrender into the shape and your breath.

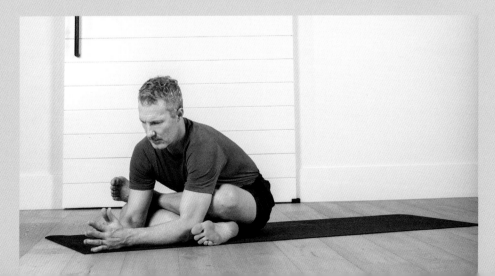

Cow Face Pose
Gomukhasana

About the Pose

This pose powerfully stretches hips, thighs, and ankles. Your legs create the shape that resembles the face of the cow, an animal revered in Indian culture.

Alignment

- Sit at the top of your mat. Extend your left leg in front of you and cross your right foot to the outside of your left thigh. Slide your left heel back by your right hip.
- Stack your knees and adjust your feet, either moving them closer to your body or away from you until you find your sweet spot.
- Press down through your seat, lift the crown of your head, and lengthen your spine.
- On your exhale, hinge at your hips and fold forward. You can stay up on your hands or move your forearms down to a block or your mat.
- Sit back up, unwind, and switch sides.

Modifications and Adaptations

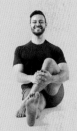

- *Modified cow face pose*: To modify, you can keep your bottom leg extended forward. Sit tall, catch the top of your shin with both hands, and fold forward to the degree that you can.

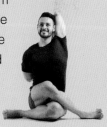

- *Cow face pose with arm bind*: For a deeper experience, add the arm bind. With your right leg on top, extend your left arm straight up to the sky, bend your elbow, and drop your left hand behind your neck. Do the opposite with your right arm, lengthen your arm to the ground, bend your elbow, and reach your right hand up your spine until your hands meet and bind. You can use a strap or towel to help make this connection. Keep the arm bind as you fold forward over your legs.

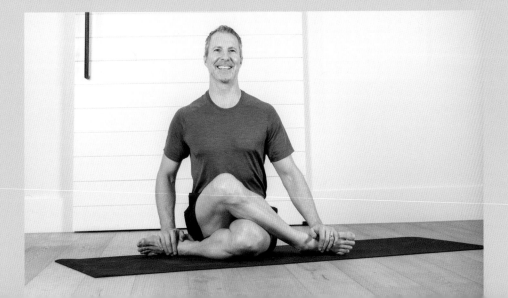

Bound Angle

Baddha Konasana

About the Pose

Bound angle helps get deep into the hips and groin. It opens and releases the muscles activated in cardio and that support you all day long through sitting and walking.

Alignment

- Be seated, bend your knees, and bring the soles of your feet together and widen your knees apart. Pull your heels close to your pelvis.
- Slide your thumbs into your arches and pull the soles of your feet, like you were opening a book.
- Root down through your seat and lift your chest up to sit tall.
- With your exhale, keep hold of your feet and fold forward and pull your chest toward your feet. Bend your elbows out to the sides and use your arms to press on your legs to get deeper into your hips and lower to the ground.
- Drop your head and breathe deeply. For a longer hold, you can extend your arms forward and turn your palms up to emphasize letting go.

Modifications and Adaptations

If your knees are high and your back is rounding, try sitting on some blankets or blocks. You can also slide your heels a few inches away from your body, keeping your feet together. Focus on maintaining the length of your spine and extension through your chest, even if that means not folding forward.

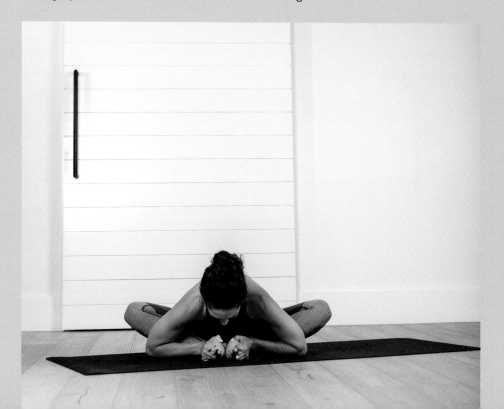

Half Splits

Ardha Hanumanasana

About the Pose

Half splits pose is a deep and juicy stretch for the hamstrings. It also stretches the thighs and groin and preps you for full splits and forward folds. Half splits is sometimes referred to as runner's lunge because it opens tightness in the legs, which helps runners.

Alignment

- Come into a low lunge position, with your right leg forward and your back knee on the ground. Tuck your back toes.
- Keep your left knee on the mat, shift your hips back over your left knee, straighten your right leg, and flex your right foot for half splits. Use blocks to support your hands if needed.
- Inhale, lift, and lengthen your chest forward.
- Exhale, hinge at your hips, and bow over your extended leg. Pull the outer edge of your front foot back, and hug your leg muscles to the bones. Allow the tension to unravel from your hamstrings and lower back as you breathe.
- To come out of the pose, shift your weight forward into your right foot, plant your hands to the top of your mat, and press back to downward-facing dog.
- Repeat low lunge and half splits on the left side.

> continued

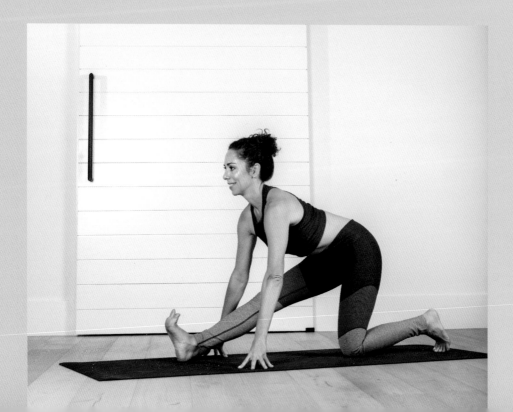

> *continued*

Modifications and Adaptations

- To deepen your fold in half splits, hold the outer edge of your right foot with your left hand and shift your left ribs toward the mat. Notice the space you open to lengthen forward and fold deeper.

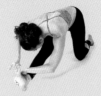

- *Full splits*: From half splits, begin to wiggle and extend your front leg forward and your back leg back until you find your edge. Roll your shoulders up and pull your arms back to open across your chest. If your legs are fully extended, you can fold forward over your front leg.

Happy Baby
Ananda Balasana

About the Pose
Happy baby opens the hips, hamstrings, and inner thighs and releases the lower back. This is a great pose to use to start your practice to gently awaken and open the hips or to use toward the end of practice to slow down your heart rate as you allow your mat and gravity to fully support you.

Alignment
- Lie on your back and hug both knees into your chest.
- Grab the outer edges of both of your feet and shine the soles of your feet toward to the sky.
- Create opposition in your legs and arms to help get deeper into your hips. Use your arms to pull your feet toward the earth and kick back into your hands.
- Rock side-to-side if that feels good.

Modifications and Adaptations
- If holding your feet is too intense, grab behind your knees and pull your thighs toward the mat.
- You can extend one or both legs straight to add hamstring stretches.
- *Half happy baby*: Bring both knees into your chest. Hold your right knee with your right hand and plant your left foot on the earth. Move your right knee toward your right armpit. Flex both feet and activate your toes. Either hold the edge of your right foot with your right hand or grab behind your knee and send your right heel up to the sky. Pull both shoulder blades onto your mat. Rest your left hand on your left hip. Use your arm strength and pull your right knee toward the earth as you kick your right foot into your right hand. This opposing action will create more opening through your hips. Bring both knees back into your chest and repeat on the other side.

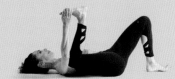

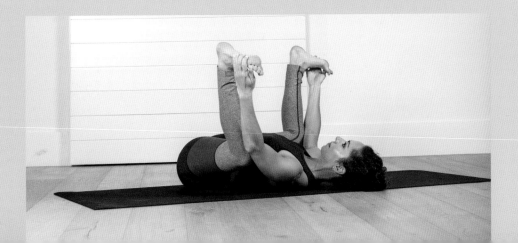

Lizard

Utthan Pristhasana

About the Pose

Lizard pose is an amazing stretch for the hip flexors, hamstrings, and quadriceps. It creates strength and opening in the legs and hips and across the pelvis. It can also be a great preparatory pose for some advanced arm balances.

Alignment

- From downward-facing dog, bring the tips of your thumbs together to touch at the center of your mat.
- Step your right foot to the outside of your right pinkie finger and lower your left knee down to the ground.
- Turn your right toes out to two o'clock, shift to the outer edge of your foot, and let your right hip open.
- Lower to your forearms or a block. If the stretch is too intense, stay lifted on your hands.
- Keep your back toes under for stability and relax your head and neck.
- Repeat on the other side (shown).

Modifications and Adaptations

- To add more challenge, lift your back knee off the ground.
- *Lizard twist*: In lizard, reach your right arm to the back of the room and open across your chest. Bend your left knee and hold your left foot with your right hand. Pull your heel toward you and stretch your quadricep. Squeeze your shoulder blades together and twist your chest up. Release your left leg slowly. Repeat on the other side.

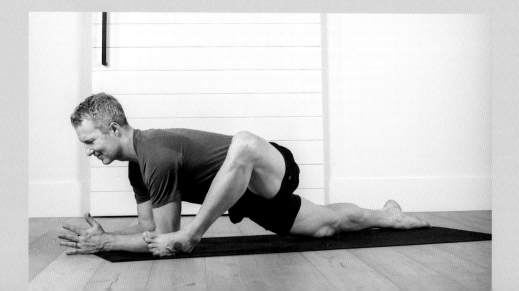

Reverse Tabletop
Ardha Purvottanasana

About the Pose

Reverse tabletop helps open the front body and create space across the heart. It counteracts the common motions of daily life that often result in tightness, tension, and rounding forward of the shoulders. It strengthens the arms, wrists, and legs and stretches the shoulders and chest. Reverse tabletop can be a less strenuous modification for backbends and is also used as a counterpose between forward folds and hip-opening poses.

Alignment

- Start seated, with your legs extended out in front of you. Bend your knees, place your feet hip-width apart, and root down through your feet.

- Plant your hands to the mat behind your hips, your fingers aiming toward the front of your mat. Press down firmly and build your foundation with your hands and your feet.

- On your inhale, lift your hips up so that your thighs and torso are parallel to the mat. Aim to align your hips with your knees and shoulders.

- Hug your shoulders in toward your spine on your back to lift your heart higher.

- If it feels good, slowly drop your head back and open your throat.

Modifications and Adaptations

Purvottanasana is the full and more advanced variation of reverse tabletop. Rather than bending your knees, keep your legs extended forward while you're seated. Press your arches together and point your toes forward. Set your hands behind your hips, with your fingers pointing toward the top of your mat. Lift your hips, keeping your legs straight and fully engaged.

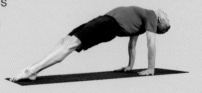

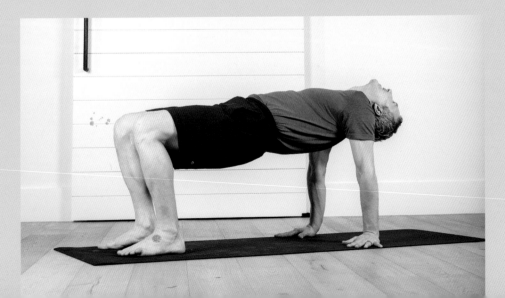

Forward Folds

Forward folds bring new energy to the whole body and vital organs as you lengthen the lower back, ribs, and torso and open the hamstrings and hips. They are intro-spective in nature, because you are turning inward to yourself, and have a calming effect on the nervous system and brain. Forward folds are cooling and help relax the mind and body at the end of class. Trust that staying true to this portion of the process creates a well-rounded workout.

When you feel your body start to resist in a fold, gently respond with your breath. Pause at the first edge you feel, bring your attention to your breath, and with time watch your edge grow. Ride your breath deeper into your fold—on every inhale, lengthen. On every exhale, fold deeper. When your mind starts to wander, simply return to your breath and tune back in to your body.

I recommend ending each practice with a seated forward fold before you roll onto your back for final rest, savasana. This helps bring all the work and experience on your mat together and brings you into your center as you honor the softer side of your power.

Seated Forward Fold
Paschimottanasana

About the Pose

Seated forward fold stretches the back, shoulders, and hamstrings. As you fold into your center, you stimulate your digestive system, liver, kidneys, and reproductive organs. This fold helps calm the brain and relieve stress and can be therapeutic for depression, fertility issues, and insomnia. Allow your breath to guide you deeper into your fold and resist the urge to force any part of the pose.

Alignment

- Sit down and extend both legs forward.
- Flex your feet, press your arches together, and activate your leg muscles.
- With your inhale, reach your arms high, hinge at your hips, and fold forward on your exhale. Catch the outer edges of both feet.
- As you inhale, lengthen your spine. With each exhale, fold deeper. Relax your neck and shoulders.
- For longer holds, release the grip of your feet and bring your hands to the mat with your palms up to emphasize letting go.

Modifications and Adaptations

Bend your knees as much as it feels good to you in this fold and lengthen through your lower back. Focus on working your ribs toward your thighs and extending your spine rather on than keeping your legs straight. You can use a strap as a connector to your feet and can sit on a block or blanket as you work to open the hamstrings.

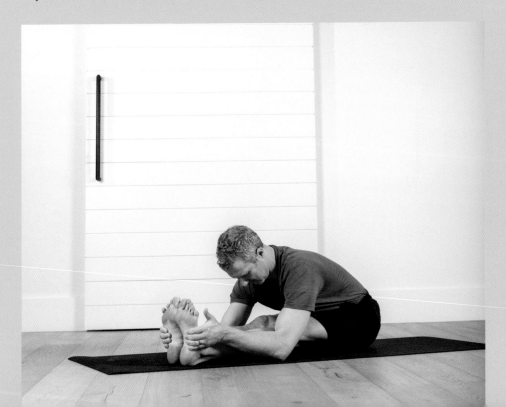

Single-Leg Forward Fold

Janu Sirsasana

About the Pose

This pose stretches and releases the calves, hamstrings, groin, back and shoulders. It flushes your digestive system, liver, and kidneys and is calming for the mind and nervous system.

Alignment

- From your seat, extend your right leg forward.
- Bend your left knee and place your left foot against your inner right thigh.
- Flex your right foot and aim all five right toes toward the ceiling.
- Anchor down through your seat.
- Inhale and reach both arms up overhead. Exhale, hinge at your hips and fold forward.
- With each inhale, lengthen. Soften into a deeper stretch with each exhale. Let your head go and relax your neck.
- Repeat on the other side (shown).

Modifications and Adaptations

- Bend the knee of your extended leg as much as you need to and lower your forehead toward your shin.
- To take it deeper, cross your left hand to catch the outside edge of your right foot and bring your left ribs down toward the mat. You can put your right fingertips back by your left hip to root and empower your torso to twist down or hold your left wrist with your right hand and create yoga mudra (thumb to your index finger) with your left hand.

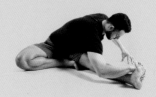

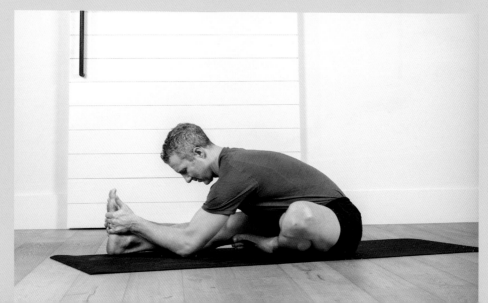

Wide-Angle Forward Fold
Upavistha Konasana

About the Pose

This wide-angle fold opens the backs of the legs and inner thighs. It stretches the lower back, strengthens the spine, and stimulates your vital organs in your abdomen.

Alignment

- Sit and separate your legs wide apart into a V shape. Flex your feet and point all your toes and your knees up to the sky.

- Place your hands to the ground in front of you, root through your seat, and lift through your chest as you inhale.

- As you exhale, slowly walk your hands forward, away from your body. Pause when you feel your back start to round or feel the first layer of resistance. Relax your neck and head and enjoy your breath.

- As you release into the pose over time, continue to walk your hands forward to find your growing edge. You can transition to your forearms, bring your chest to the ground, or grab the outsides of your feet.

Modifications and Adaptations

If you are working with tighter hamstrings, sit up on a blanket or block. You can also place a block under your head to support you in the fold.

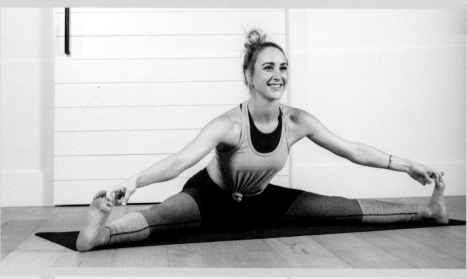

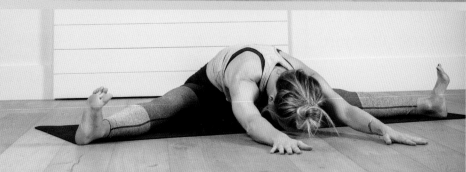

Final Rest

How often do you find that you are in a rush? In a world where everything moves fast, yoga helps us slow down, go within, pause, and restore our power. As we've learned to do more in less time, many people are finding it harder not only to slow down but also sleep. In 2013, the Centers for Disease Control reported that over 9 million Americans were taking a sleep aid to help them fall and stay asleep at night, and it estimated that millions more were using over-the-counter sedatives. These drugs and other numbing agents, whether it's a couple of glasses of wine or some low-quality television, are ways of reaching outside of ourselves to slow down and shut down the body and mind. In our quest to do more and be more, we can go so fast that it can feel counterintuitive to add a practice of active rest. However, there is tremendous power in doing things differently, and at the end of a power yoga practice, we take time to choose rest, simply being and not doing.

The final pose in every yoga practice is the most important pose. Yogis have known for centuries that there is power in the rest, so they included corpse pose, savasana, at the end of every practice. At the end of your time on your mat, take 5 to 10 minutes to lie still in deep rest. In this quiet space of rest and surrender, you allow the benefits from your practice to integrate into your physical, energetic, and emotional bodies. Savasana is where all your work comes together and takes root within. This integration time is essential for getting the most out of your practice.

As you lie on your mat in savasana, you reap the many benefits of this pose. Final rest teaches surrender and allows your yoga practice to settle into you. Other benefits of savasana are:

Relaxation

Trains you to be conscious and tension-free

Reduces stress and fatigue

Allows for integration of your practice physically and energetically

Brings the body and mind into balance

Increases self-awareness

Gives the experience of oneness, peace, and union

> How beautiful it is to do nothing and then rest afterward.
>
> Spanish proverb

In savasana, you get to practice surrendering all effort. Surrender is the opposite of giving up your power. It's an act of complete trust and faith

Try adding more rest and purposeful pauses into other parts of your day. Take rest between meetings or after lunch. Go for a walk without your phone, lie down in your office and rest your legs up on the wall, close your eyes for a few deep breaths, and calm your mind whenever time allows. These poses and practices are not just for your yoga mat. Rest allows you to integrate, assimilate, and use all that happens in your life. There is power in taking the time to let your practice of life land within you. When you are rested, you can bring that much more to your life, workouts, friends, family, and everything you do. Rest opens you to a more powerful way of being.

that all is well, that you are fully supported, and that you are connected divinely to and one with the energy that unites all of life. For these few minutes in your day while you are completely free from responsibility, you can leave stress behind and allow yourself to recharge. All you have to do is relax and receive the gifts from your practice and the rejuvenating benefits from your rest. Be still and let your transformation and learning settle into you. This purposeful pause brings you back to your natural state and gives body, mind, and spirit chance to settle and come together. The more you practice this complete surrender, the more you access the powerful benefits of rest and relaxation to use in the rest of your life.

When your final pose, final rest, is complete, keep your eyes closed and gently begin to reawaken. Rub your thumbs over the pads of your fingers and wiggle your toes. Slowly roll your wrists and ankles out. When you are ready, bring your knees to your chest and wrap your arms around your shins. In this small ball, gently roll onto your right or left side, whatever side is calling you. Pause here for a moment of gratitude while your energy is still soft and inward. With your eyes closed, silently give thanks to your body for working for you so willingly. Acknowledge the people and circumstances in your life that have made it possible for you to practice yoga, from the coworkers supporting you in your life's work, to your partner for holding it down at home. And of course, honor your efforts on the mat and acknowledge yourself for doing the work. Stay here as long as it feels right.

When you are ready, with your eyes still closed, gently press yourself up to a seated position with your ankles crossed. Unite your palms at heart center in anjali mudra. In this meditative seat, scan your body and mind and notice what's available. What's possible after you've been in a practice of consciously creating your breath, moving with purpose, and aligning with your higher intention? How do you feel now? And how can

> To the mind that is still, the whole universe surrenders.
>
> Lao Tzu

End Powerfully

Don't rush or skip the cool-down or savasana. I find that a lot of power yoga teachers spend most of the class strengthening and turning up the energy of the class and then leave out time for finishing poses and restoration. This is a disservice to your students since it does not give them a complete practice. Students come to yoga to realign themselves—body, mind, and spirit. Even the most athletic students are looking for what yoga offers beyond just a workout. Asana and meditation switch on the parasympathetic nervous system, which calms the body and the brain, stimulates immune system, keeps the endocrine system healthy, and frees your vital energy to flow. This brings the body back to equilibrium. Hold space for your students to rest and digest their practice. These final poses give everyone a chance to turn inward and let go. Plan your class and manage your time to ensure a powerful ending and bring your best to this part of class. This section is a great time to support students individually with modifications, props, and hands-on assists. Lower the lights in the room, play music that facilitates turning inward, and hold space for silence before you close the class. End your classes with purpose and power.

you carry this forward into the rest of your life? Yoga comes to life when we bring it to life. Take a few quiet moments to reflect on how you want to share and expand your power with others and in your life. With your hands still at heart center, you can bookend your practice by chanting Om three times.

Slowly lift your prayer hands to your forehead, in front of the third eye. Seal the insights and wisdom from your body into your mind. We end by bowing the head and heart toward the earth and saying, "Namaste." *Namaste* means (or translates to) "the light in me honors the light within you." This gesture is a deep form of respect for the practice of yoga, for your body and for the knowledge that has been shared and passed down to you. In a class, namaste is shared as a symbol of respect and gratitude to close the class. The teacher bows to the students and to their own teachers and lineage. In return, it gives the students an opportunity to thank and honor the teacher for guidance and energy. When we acknowledge and appreciate each other, we see and expand the divine light within us and that unites us.

Final Rest
Savasana

About the Pose

Final rest, also known as corpse pose, is the purposeful rest at the end of every practice. This is the one pose that should never be skipped. Savasana allows your nerves to recuperate, your organs become passive, your body to surrender all effort, and your mind to let go of responsibility and relax. This rest allows your efforts on the mat to settle into your body, integrate into the nervous system, and become you. Gradually, this leads to greater detachment and feeling rejuvenated and more alive. Corpse pose allows you to leave behind what you no longer need and let the excess die. When you come up from your rest, you have a blank canvas for a new beginning.

Alignment

- Lie on your back with your legs extended long and your arms by your sides.
- Relax your legs completely, and let your feet splay out to the sides. Take up your space.
- Turn your palms face up as a symbol that you are open and available to receive the benefits from your practice.
- Close your eyes, let go of your ujjayi breath, and return to your natural breath.
- Surrender all your muscles, all your effort, and come into an active rest. Your body and mind are still conscious.

Modifications and Adaptations

If you feel pain in your lower back, bend your knees, place your feet on the floor, and bring your knees together.

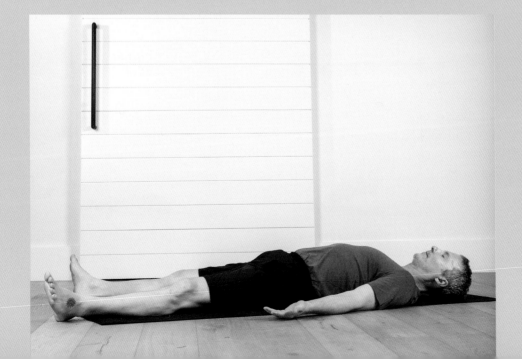

Cool-Down Sequences

The cool-down is your opportunity to stretch, open, and strengthen in a different way. Relax into these poses and allow your body and mind to rest and recover. As with everything in power yoga, the energy that you create in your experience is more important than the specific poses. For your cool-down, consider the energy of your overall practice and peak poses, how to stretch and release muscles activated in your flow, and which poses will open and empower you. This is also a great place to give yourself a little extra love and pay attention to areas of your body that have been calling out for more care. Rest is essential to thrive and heal.

Here are some suggestions for cool-down sequences. Allow your breath to guide you into your body in these longer, deeper holds. Be in the practice of acceptance and letting go.

5-Minute Cool-Down

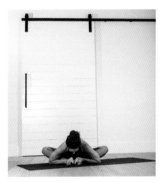

1 Bound angle for 10 breaths
(page 228)

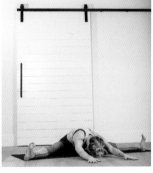

2 Wide-angle forward fold
for 10 breaths
(page 237)

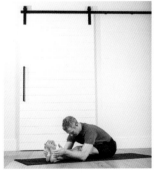

3 Seated forward fold
for 10 breaths
(page 235)

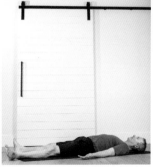

4 Final rest for two minutes
or more
(page 241)

10-Minute Cool-Down

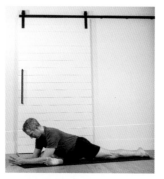

1 Half pigeon for 15 breaths
on each side
(page 224)

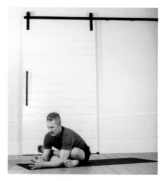

2 Double pigeon for
10 breaths each side
(page 226)

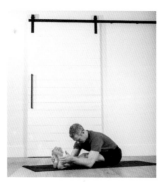

3 Seated forward fold
for 10 breaths
(page 235)

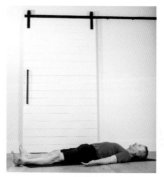

4 Final rest for 4 minutes
or more
(page 241)

15-Minute Cool-Down

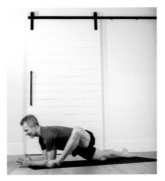

1 Lizard for 10 breaths
(page 232)

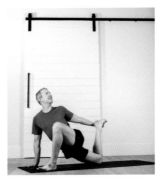

2 Lizard twist for
10 breaths each side
(page 232)

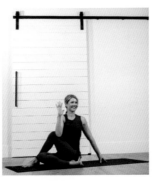

3 Seated twist for 5 breaths
each side
(page 157)

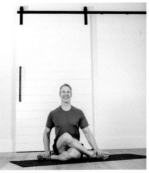

4 Cow face pose for
15 breaths each side
(page 227)

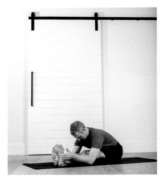

5 Seated forward fold
for 20 breaths
(page 235)

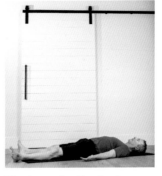

6 Final rest for 5 minutes
or more
(page 241)

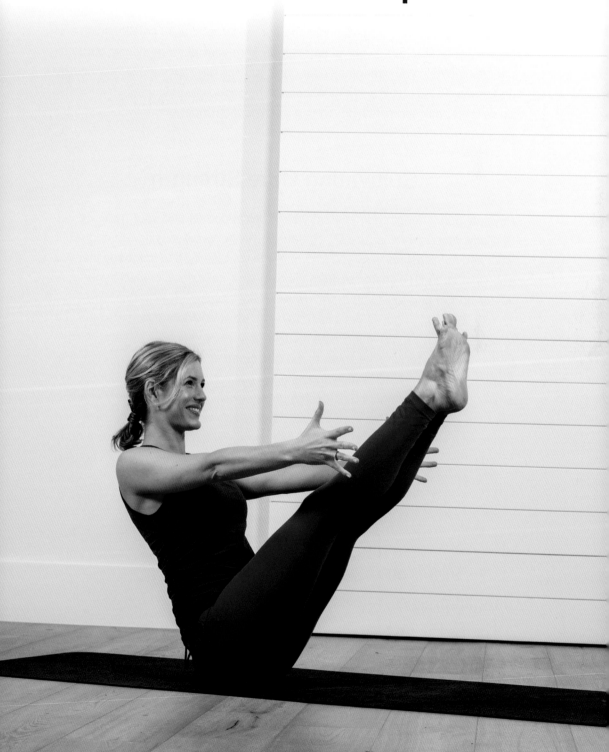

CHAPTER 8
Core Strength Poses and Sequences

The core is the power center within the body, and core strength affects every pose. Powerful abdominal muscles support your everyday movements, improve your posture, stabilize your lower back, and support your overall health and vitality. In yoga, strong abs create more efficient movements and power within every pose. Outside of yoga, strong abs allow you to move through your other workouts with greater stability and efficiency.

The poses and sequences in this chapter will target crucial core muscles and improve your strength. Every pose extends from your physical center out in all directions. When you strengthen your core, you can open all sorts of new energy and power. These poses and sequences can be added into your practice within the power and peak segments, or you can practice them independently for a shorter core-focused practice.

Cultivating Core Strength

Physical core strength comes from your lower abdomen and your navel center. Similarly, your core values are what guides you in the rest of your life—through your work and relationships, how you show up with your family, and the foods that you eat. Core strength also comes from aligning your daily decisions with your core values and what is most important to you.

Your low belly, or gut, is like a second brain. It's now widely understood that the microbiome in the gut is much more than just part of the digestive system. Millions of neurons are found in the lining of the gut, creating a complex ecosystem that responds to external stimulation and reflects your inner environment. Your second brain doesn't think in thoughts, it communicates with sensation. Have you heard the term *gut check*? That's when you check your commitments, priorities, and values at a visceral level before you take action. You tap into your physical body for communication and listen to your inner wisdom for guidance on what's coming up in your life and how to respond.

> Yoga is an internal practice. The rest is just a circus.
>
> Sri K. Pattabhi Jois

When you're faced with a decision, take a breath, close your eyes, and listen to the energetic response from your lower abdomen, your core. Do you feel nervousness, butterflies, a sense of caution, or excitement? When you start to flex these muscles within your core—both physical and energetic—you build more connection to your inner guidance system and intuition. The more you listen, the more you empower your inner wisdom and your mind-body connection. Start to drop out of your thinking mind and tune in to your gut for direction and guidance.

Your core center is the space of the solar plexus, the energetic center that embodies the strength and power of the sun. It is important to listen here for passion and excitement when you do your gut check. When something is really calling for your attention, you'll feel it in your gut. Think about how you've felt physically when you've gone out on a first date and know you've met someone special; during the first part of a project, when you get the sense that you're on to something great; or when you're training for a race or competition and you make it over a mental or physical block that takes your skill to a new level. These breakthroughs and turning points come with a rush of new energy. This is where tapas in yoga philosophy comes into play. You'll feel the zest, burning desire, or passion to move something forward. This inner calling is communication from your spirit.

Here are a few questions to consider when you are building your core strength. When you ask yourself these questions, try placing both hands on your low belly, close your eyes, and tune in to your inner guidance from your core.

What do I feel? Can I put a label on these sensations?

What do I really want to create in this situation?

Does this feel in alignment with my true self?

Is this creating the energy I want to feel?

Is this action in alignment with my core values?

When you move from inner wisdom and feel good in your body, your confidence will soar both on and off the mat. You can start to lean on and trust your inner wisdom—your body's inherent intelligence. This deep source of inner strength allows you to move through the world with more grace and ease and puts you in touch with your personal power.

Core Poses

In these poses, we'll focus on working from the center of your body and developing your core strength. Bring your attention to toning and strengthening your abdominal muscles as well as moving from your center in all transitions. Moving from your core creates total body integration and keeps you aligned with your rhythmic breath and bandhas. Tune in to your inner guidance and breath to know how far to go in each pose. Use your exhales to hug into your core center and stoke your inner flame. Use the light from your inhales to expand from the inside out.

> The success of yoga does not lie in the ability to perform postures but in how it positively changes the way we live our life and our relationships.
>
> T.K.V. Desikachar

Boat
Navasana

About the Pose

Boat pose strengthens your core and creates balance and whole-body integration. It tones the abdominal wall and hip flexors and stabilizes and supports the lower back. Pull your power into your center and lift your sails high.

Alignment

- Be seated and plant both feet on the ground with your knees bent. Sit up tall and balance on your seat.

- Hook your hands behind your knees and lift your heels to knee level or extend your heels up and forward. Press the arches together and spread your toes to activate your feet.

- You can keep your hands behind your knees for support, or extend your hands forward and spread your fingers. Draw your upper arm bones back and broaden your chest.

- Engage your lower abdomen and lift your heart high.

- To come out of the pose, cross your ankles, roll over your feet, and step back to plank pose or downward-facing dog.

Modifications and Adaptations

- *Full boat with straight legs*: To intensify this pose, extend your heels high, and reach your arms forward. Activate your feet and fan your toes open.

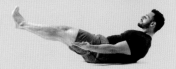

- *Supported boat*: Place your hands behind your knees, bend your knees, and lift your shins parallel to the ground or touch your toes to the mat. Engage your lower abdomen and lift your chest up and open.

- *Low boat*: Lower down until your legs and upper back hover above the floor in a line. Extend your arms forward and keep your back broad.

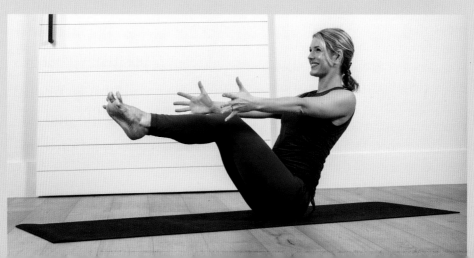

Scissor Crunches

About the Pose

Scissor crunches tone and strengthen your entire abdominal wall, build heat, and focus your energy.

Alignment

- Lie on your back, extend both heels to the sky, and flex both feet. Ignite your legs and hug your muscles to the bones.

- Extend both arms to the sky and unite your palms, like an arrow. Lower your right leg to hover 6 to 12 inches off the ground.

- On your exhale, lift your chest and reach your arms to the outside of your left knee. With your exhales, hug your lower abdomen toward the earth, lift your chest and shoulders, pulse up, and lower on your inhales. Complete 10 or more, then transition to the other side.

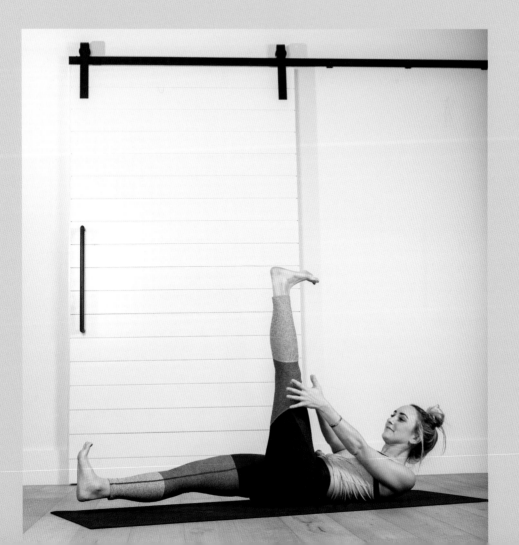

Scissor Kicks

About the Pose

Scissor kicks tone and strengthen your core and build integration and coordination of your upper body and lower body.

Alignment

- Lie on your back, extend both heels to the sky, and flex both feet. Ignite your legs and hug your muscles to the bones.
- Lengthen your arms along the side of your body and press your palms flat on the ground.
- Lower your left leg so your heel hovers 6 inches off the earth.
- Fully extend on your exhales and transition to the other side on your inhales to move with one breath per movement.

Modifications and Adaptations

To modify, place your hands with the palms down underneath your seat to slightly elevate your hips and support your lower back.

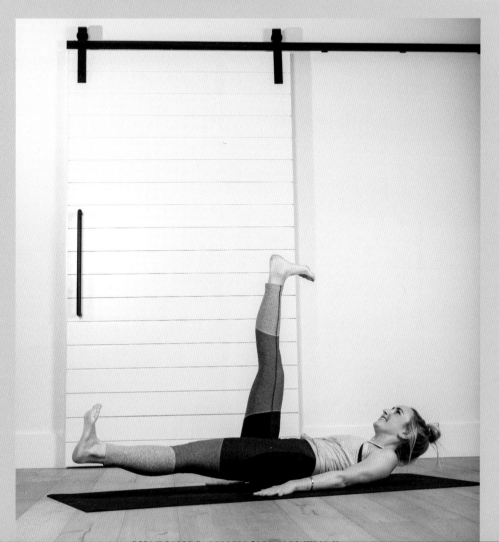

Plank Curls

About the Pose

Plank curls are core-building transitions that emphasize moving from your core strength and center. There are three main variations as you shift forward and ignite your core.

Alignment

- Start in either downward-facing dog or high plank.
- On your exhale, shift forward and touch your right knee to your right triceps. Engage your core and lift your knee high up toward your armpit.
- With your inhale, press your right leg up and back to a down dog split.
- As you exhale, shift forward and cross your right knee to your left elbow. Lift your belly and squeeze your obliques (shown).
- Inhale, extend, and press back to a down dog split.
- On your exhale, bring your knee forward toward your nose, arch your upper back.
- Inhale, return to a down dog split, and lower your right foot down.
- Switch to your left side and then repeat for a second set on each side.

Modifications and Adaptations

- Instead of starting in downward-facing dog or high plank, you can modify and build core strength with curls in tabletop pose.
- *Plank waves:* From downward-facing dog, on your inhale, extend forward into high plank. On your exhale, lift your hips up and back into downward-facing dog. Continue to move with one breath per movement to create the wavelike motions of expanding forward to plank as you breathe in and pulling back to down dog as you breathe out. Initiate the movements of this rhythmic flow from your core.

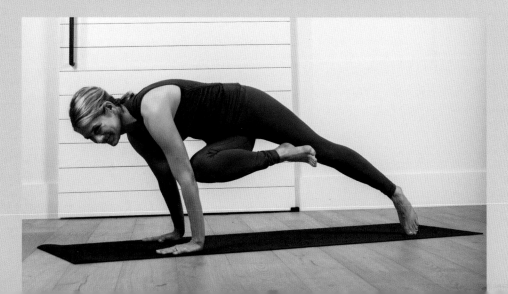

Bicycles

About the Pose

These abdominal twists access the deep core muscles and fire up your obliques, the muscles that help rotate your body.

Alignment

- Lie on your back and create a 90-degree angle with your legs. Flex your feet.
- Interlace your hands behind your head, open your elbows, and keep your chest broad.
- Before you lift your chest, activate your core and pull the abdominal muscles in.
- Extend your right leg out long and keep your left knee bent. With your exhale, lift your right elbow to your left knee. Pedal your legs, and use your exhales to cross your opposite elbow to meet the opposite knee. Transition to your other side on your inhales. One leg goes in as the other leg goes out.

Modifications and Adaptations

If lifting your chest creates strain in your neck, modify by only using the actions in your legs.

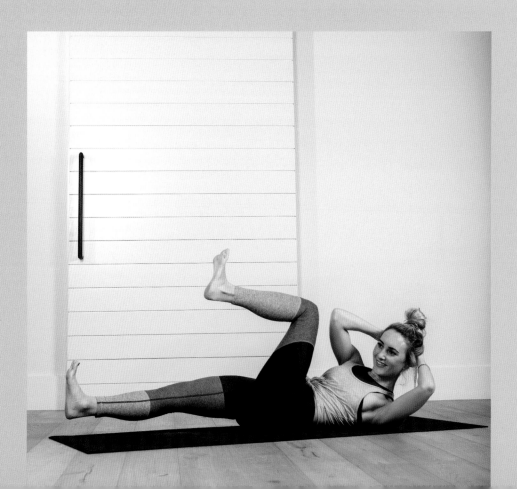

Crow Crunches

About the Pose

Crow pose strengthens the upper body and core and leads to balance and lightness when done on the hands. On the back, it creates serious ab strengthening.

Alignment

- Lie down on your back and stretch out long. Lift your heels 6 inches off the ground and reach your arms overhead.

- Engage your center, pull your belly button to your spine, and firm your legs.

- Take a deep breath in. With your exhale, round up, curl into a tight ball and come into crow on your back. Hug your knees against the back of your arms, close to your armpits, and hollow out your midsection. Press the arches of your feet together and awaken your toes to ignite the power line up to your core.

- Repeat these actions, moving one breath per movement, extending on your inhales and contracting on your exhales.

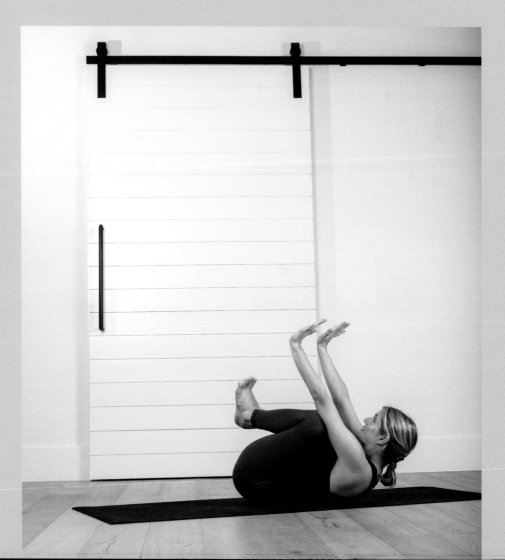

Core Sequences

These sequences will stoke your inner fire and create cleansing heat through your entire body. You can practice these sequences independently or add them in after warm-ups and power sequences to build heat. The sequences are poses that specifically target the core and include some foundational poses from previous chapters. Together, these elements create a core-centered, well-rounded sequence.

5-Minute Core Sequence

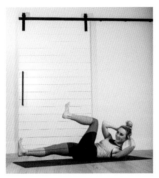

1 Bicycles for 10 each side (20 total breaths)
   (page 252)

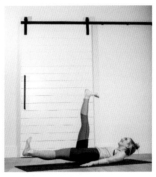

2 Scissor kicks for 30 kicks (30 breaths)
   (page 250)

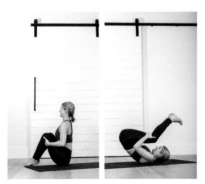

3 Rock 'n' roll 3 times (3 breaths)
   (page 74)

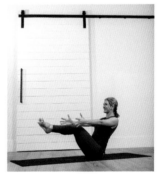

4 Boat for 10 breaths
   (page 248)

5 Transition: cross your ankles, roll over your feet, and make your way into downward-facing dog

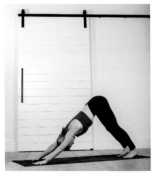
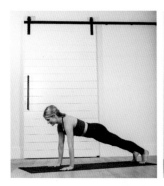
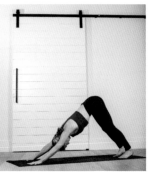

6 Downward-facing dog
for 5 breaths
(page 80)

7 Plank waves for 5 breaths
(page 251)

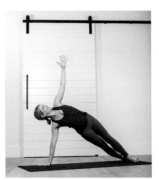
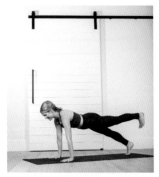

8 High plank for 5 breaths
(page 85)

9 Three-point plank for 3 breaths
(page 86)

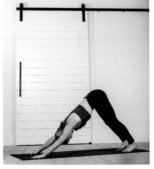

10 Side plank with crossed
ankles for 5 breaths
(page 190)

11 Downward-facing dog
for 5 breaths
(page 80)

12 Repeat on other side

10-Minute Core Sequence

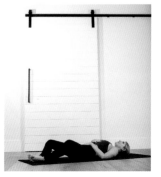

1 Reclined bound angle
for 5 breaths
(page 68)

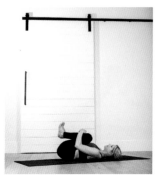

2 Knees-to-chest for
3 breaths
(page 73)

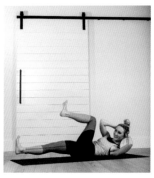

3 Bicycles for 20 rounds
or more
(page 252)

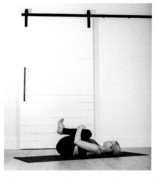

4 Knees-to-chest for 3 breaths
(page 73)

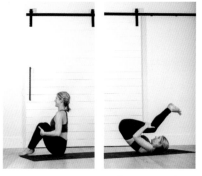

5 Rock 'n' roll 5 times (5 breaths)
(page 74)

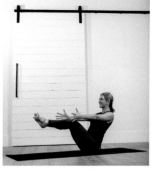

6 Boat for 5 breaths
(page 248)

7 Transition: cross your ankles, roll over your feet, and make your way
into downward-facing dog

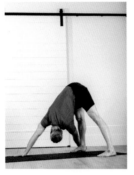

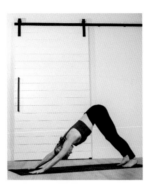

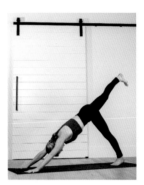

8 Wide down dog twists for 5 breaths each side (page 160)

9 Downward-facing dog for 5 breaths (page 80)

10 Inhale: down dog splits (page 81)

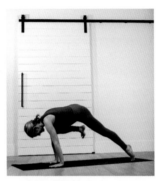

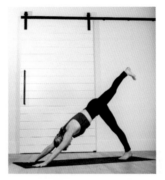

11 Exhale: plank curl to right triceps (page 251)

12 Inhale: down dog splits (page 81)

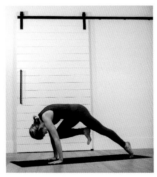

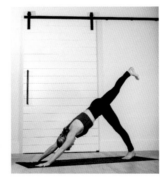

13 Exhale: plank curl to nose (page 251)

14 Inhale: down dog splits (page 81)

> continued

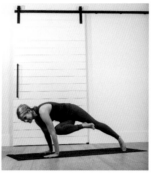

15 Exhale: knee to the left triceps, then kick into fallen triangle
(page 251 and 191)

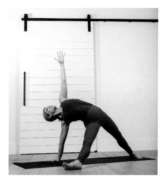

16 Inhale: fallen triangle, lift your left arm
(page 191)

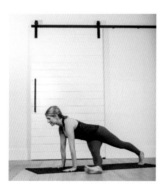

17 Exhale: fallen triangle, reground through your left hand
(page 191)

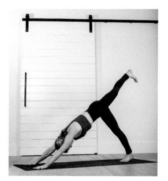

18 Inhale: down dog splits
(page 81)

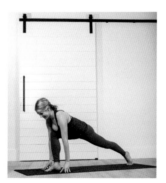

19 Exhale: step your right foot forward into a lunge
(page 125)

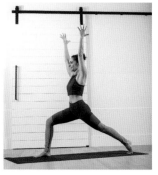

20 Crescent lunge for 5 breaths
(page 124)

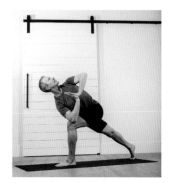

21 Crescent twist for 5 breaths
(page 155)

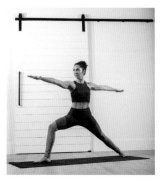

22 Warrior II for 5 breaths
(page 117)

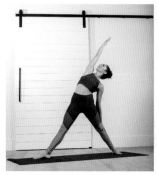

23 Reverse triangle for 5 breaths
(page 122)

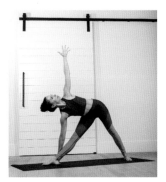

24 Triangle for 5 breaths
(page 121)

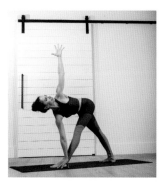

25 Twisting triangle for 5 breaths
(page 158)

> continued

26 Vinyasa (page 98): first time through, 5 breaths per pose;
repeat one more time at one breath per movement

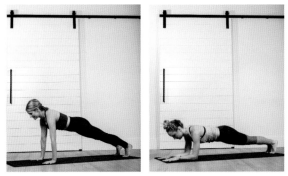

27 High plank to forearm plank for 5 rounds
(page 85 and 192)

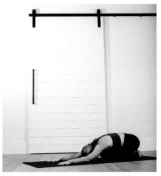

28 Child's pose for 5 breaths
or more
(page 63)

15-Minute Core Sequence

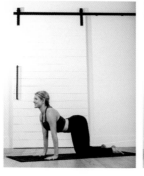

1 Cat and cow for 5 rounds
(page 66)

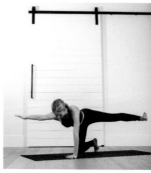

2 Extended tabletop
for 5 breaths
(page 65)

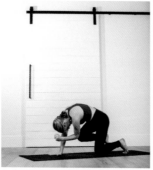

3 Tabletop crunches
for 5 rounds each side
(page 65)

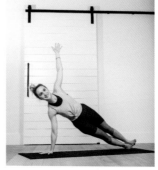

4 Awkward airplane
for 5 breaths each side
(page 65)

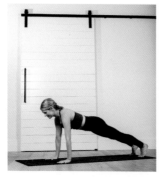

5 High plank for 5 breaths
(page 85)

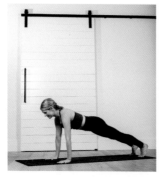

6 Side plank for 5 breaths
each side
(page 190)

> continued

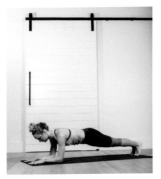

7 Forearm plank for 5 breaths
(page 192)

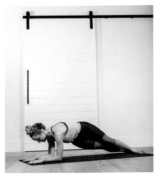

8 Forearm plank with heel
twists for 10 rounds
(page 192)

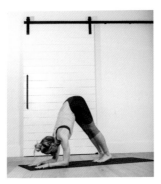

9 Dolphin for 5 breaths
(page 199)

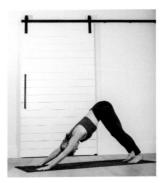

10 Downward-facing dog
for 5 breaths
(page 80)

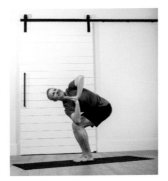

11 Chair twist for 5 breaths on each
side and one breath to center
between sides, then transition to
the top of the mat into chair
(page 153)

12 Vinyasa
(page 98)

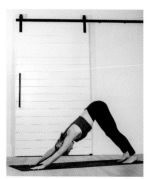

13 Downward-facing dog
for 5 breaths
(page 80)

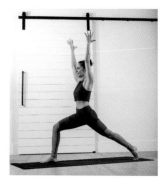

14 Crescent lunge for 5 breaths
(page 124)

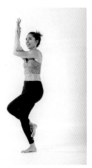

15 Eagle for 5 breaths
(page 140)

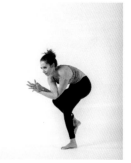

16 Nested eagle for 5 breaths
(page 141)

> continued

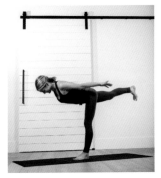

17 Airplane for 5 breaths
(page 150)

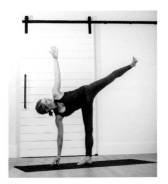

18 Half moon for 5 breaths
(page 148)

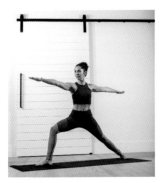

19 Warrior II for 5 breaths
(page 117)

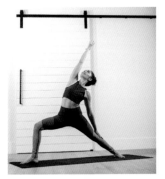

20 Reverse warrior for 5 breaths
(page 118)

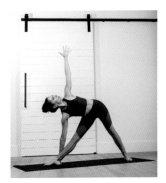

21 Triangle for 5 breaths
(page 121)

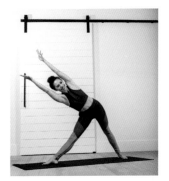

22 Extended-arm triangle
for 5 breaths
(page 122)

23 Vinyasa (page 98) and repeat on other side (first time through, 5 breaths per pose, repeat two more times at one breath per movement)

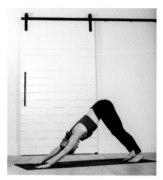

24 Downward-facing dog for 5 breaths
(page 80)

25 Transition: walk halfway up the mat and sit, or hop to the top of the mat and make your way into a seat

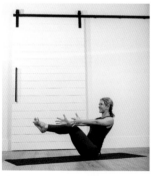

26 Boat for 10 breaths
(page 248)

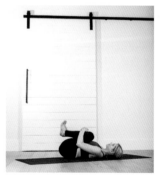

27 Knees-to-chest for 3 breaths
(page 73)

> continued

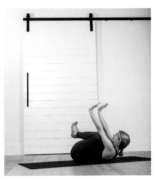

28 Crow crunches
for 10 rounds
(page 253)

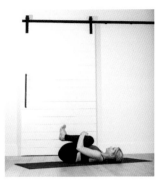

29 Knees-to-chest for 3 breaths
(page 73)

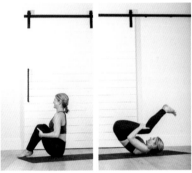

30 Rock 'n' roll 3 times (3 breaths)
(page 74)

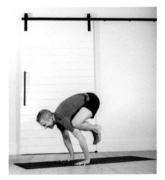

31 Crow for 5 to 10 breaths
(page 187)

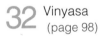

32 Vinyasa
(page 98)

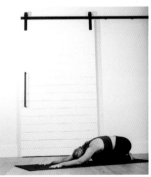

33 Child's pose for 5 breaths or more
(page 63)

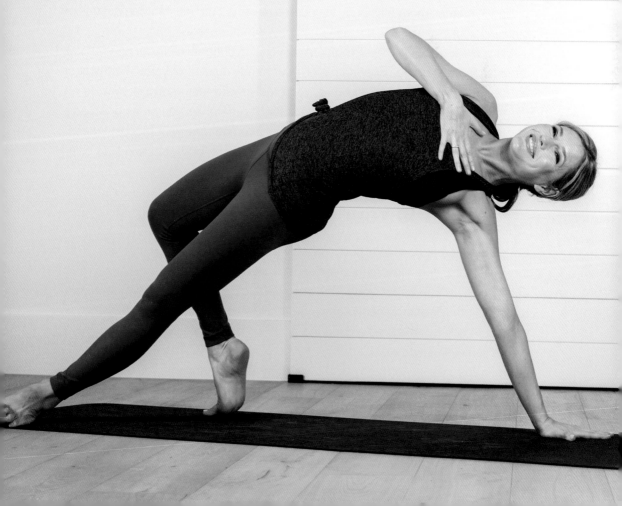

CHAPTER 9

Upper-Body Strength Sequences

Yoga is an incredible way to build upper-body strength and tone and sculpt all the muscles in the arms, chest, and back. The poses in these upper-body strength-building sequences will help you cultivate long, lean muscles in your arms and flexibility in your shoulders and chest.

When I lift weights, I can create muscle mass quickly. This can be beneficial, but it also comes with limits. I tend to carry stress and tension in my shoulders and neck already, and I've also had injuries that limit my mobility. For me, adding mass through lifting can feel constrictive, leaving me feeling more tense across my chest, shoulders, and neck. It wasn't until I committed to power yoga—and using my own body weight to build strength—that I started to see results that were unique to my own body and practice. I could build strength and muscle definition as well as flexibility and openness.

Your body weight will help you identify the areas that will be most beneficial for you to both strengthen and release. You'll get direct feedback from your body of where you are overworked or atrophied—it happens to everyone because we all have life patterns and actions that we repeat every day. Your body weight is usually a little more than you would pick up with weights, and body weight exercises are easier on your joints. Additionally, the integrated actions of pushing away and pulling in creates more efficiency in your movements that you can carry into your other workouts.

Many of the poses in power yoga are built on the foundation of your hands. How often as an adult do you spend time on your hands outside of yoga? For most of us, it's not that often, if ever. In power yoga, downward-facing dog is considered the "home base" pose and the shape that you return to. As you press down and pull up through your hands and arms, you activate and tone your biceps, triceps, shoulders, and upper back. Every muscle in your upper body is utilized in power yoga.

What Is Your Upper Body Saying?

Body language is how your body communicates nonverbally through your posture, gestures, and movements. It happens all the time, both consciously and unconsciously. The upper body—the shoulders, chest, and arms—surround and protect the major energy center of the heart. How your body holds this space, or how your body is structured around the heart, communicates volumes about you before you even say a word.

When you create neutral alignment, the alignment of tadasana, you open across the chest and brighten from the inside out. Remember that tadasana is the blueprint for all yoga poses, and you build tadasana in your upper body by lengthening the sides of your body from your hips to your shoulders, and drawing your upper arm bones onto your back. Hug the lower tips of your shoulder blades toward your spine, soften your thoracic spine in, and lift your chest up. By working from the blueprint in every pose, you start to hold your body in a way that opens you to more life force energy to flow across your chest and through your heart center, which can be incredibly calming and healing.

By opening and strengthening the structure and muscles of your upper body, you will automatically shift and elevate your energy. This outer adjustment affects your inner alignment. Your body and being start to attract matching energies of people, places, and opportunities. When you do the work of taking ownership of your energy and actions, you'll feel more uplifted and so will everyone around you. Let your body and your asana reflect the energy you want to feel all the time, everywhere.

The body and mind are so connected that just thinking about a situation affects your posture. Most of the time when we are focused on what is going well and is working for us, we sit up tall and light up from the inside out. However, when we focus on what doesn't feel good or where we feel unsatisfied, the body responds with the shoulders collapsing and rounding forward. Your body contracts, and your energy closes off. This becomes even more dramatic when we have experienced trauma or heartache or are living in lower-level energies for an extended amount of time. When the shoulders round forward, it is a primal, animalistic posture. It comes from needing to protect the vital organs and heart. Think about a pet dog walking on all fours. When the dog is challenged or threatened, it tenses across the chest, pulls back on its hind legs, and is ready to protect or fight. When the same dog feels safe and loved, he rolls onto his back and allows you to pet his belly and chest. He opens his body and takes down his guard.

This also happens with us. If your body signals that you are guarded, the same reservations will be reflected back to you. How you create your body creates your reality. The physical and energetic work as one.

The good news is that the body is easily adaptable and malleable, and it's not fixed. When you practice power yoga and create optimal alignment in your body repeatedly, you open yourself up to new energy and new opportunity. As you practice creating your postures in ways that align with how want to feel now, you can start to unwind old holding patterns and release limiting beliefs. You start to embody the energy of something greater than what you've experienced before. Your body begins to return to your natural, neutral posture and communicates that you are open, available, and ready for what's possible now.

In this simple exercise, you'll reflect on a situation in your life and witness how your body responds. The more you can tune in to what your upper body is saying, the more insight and information you'll access to use in your life.

Come into a comfortable seat and close your eyes. Take a deep breath in and feel your breath filling your lungs completely. Open your mouth and exhale all your air. Keep your eyes closed, and recall a situation in your life that isn't going as well as you'd like. Think of a situation right now in your life where you are feeling stuck, resistant, or unsatisfied. It could be within a relationship, not achieving the results you want with a project, or something within your yoga practice. The situation will be unique to you, but the energy is familiar to us all. Where are you feeling a sense of resistance or struggle in your life right now? See the details in your mind.

As you think about this situation and the circumstances contributing to this situation, notice how it feels in your body. Specifically, how does it feel in your upper body? Notice how your body embraces this situation when you think about it.

Take another deep breath in to fill your upper chest. Open your mouth and exhale all your air to clear the slate and shift your focus.

Now, recall something going well in your life. It could be a relationship, something with your work, or an activity that brings you joy. What are the circumstances that contribute to you feeling satisfied and inspired? What are the factors that have impacted you? As you focus on this situation, notice how your body responds. How does this feel in your upper body?

Take a deep breath in, and open your mouth and exhale all your air. What did you notice as you reflected on your two different situations? When you felt resistant, your body was saying no to something. When you felt inspired, something within you was saying, "Yes, more of this." How did it feel and how did your body respond? As yogis, we use our bodies as instruments and the postures increase our sensitivity—both within our bodies and to the world around us. Listen to your body language, both in yoga poses and in your life, to better align yourself to you power.

When the body and mind work together to uplift your energy, the results multiply. Create your posture as a living practice and make your highest intention physical. Align your body to create more purpose and power, on and off the mat.

Upper-Body Sequences

These sequences will emphasize both strengthening and opening your upper body. To maximize your power in these poses, firmly press down through the knuckles of your hands and establish a solid foundation. As you press down, also pull up through your hands, arms, and shoulders to create stability and integration. These sequences will utilize every muscle in your upper body and will sculpt your biceps, triceps, shoulders, and upper back.

Pay close attention to the signals from your body that call you to create your optimal blueprint of tadasana in order to stay strong and open. When the shoulders round forward in a yoga pose, that's a cue from the body that you've gone too far or that you've shifted out of alignment.

These sequences are powerful to practice on their own, but you can also add them in after warm-ups and power sequences target your upper body. You can also thread the poses in these sequences into your overall practice to bring more focus to the upper body.

> Put your heart, mind, and soul into even your smallest acts. This is the secret of success.
>
> Swami Sivananda

5-Minute Upper-Body Sequence

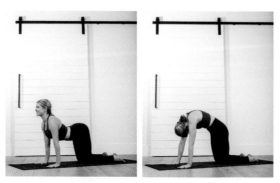

1 Cat and cow for 5 rounds
(page 66)

> continued

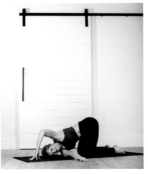

2 Thread the needle for
5 breaths each side
(page 72)

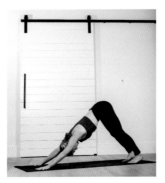

3 Downward-facing dog for
5 breaths
(page 80)

4 Transition: walk hands to the back of the mat

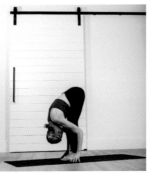

5 Standing forward fold
for 5 breaths
(page 83)

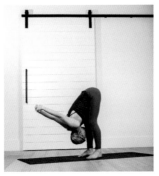

6 Standing forward fold
with a bind for 5 breaths
(page 83)

7 Transition: walk hands to the front of the mat

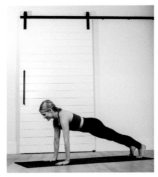

8 High plank for 5 breaths
(page 85)

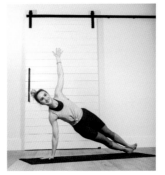

9 Side plank on the right side
for 5 breaths
(page 190)

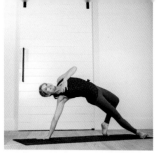

10 Wild thing for 5 breaths
(page 191)

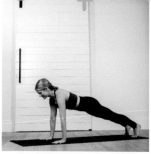

11 High plank for 5 breaths
(page 85)

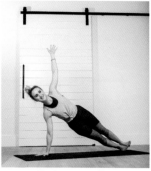

12 Side plank on the left side
for 5 breaths
(page 190)

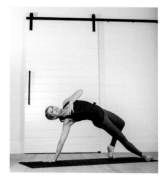

13 Wild thing for 5 breaths
(page 191)

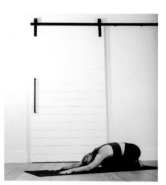

14 Child's pose for 5 breaths
or more
(page 63)

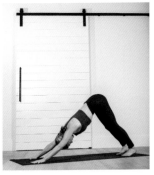

1 Downward-facing dog
for 5 breaths
(page 80)

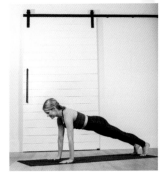

2 High plank for 5 breaths
(page 85)

3 Transition: lower down to the floor for 5 counts (5 breaths).

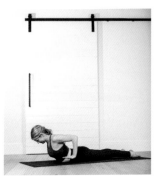

4 Low cobra with palms
lifted, 3 times with 3
rounds of breath
(page 89)

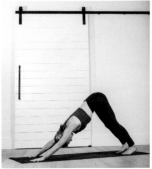

5 Downward-facing dog
for 5 breaths
(page 80)

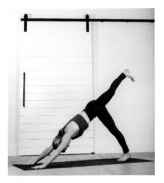

6 Inhale: down dog splits
(page 81)

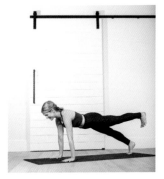

7 Exhale and inhale:
three-point plank
(page 86)

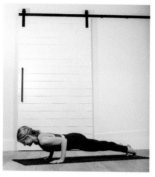

8 Exhale: low plank
(page 87)

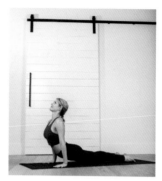

9 Inhale: upward-facing dog
(page 88)

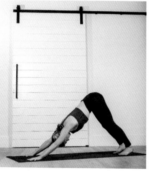

10 Exhale: downward-facing dog
(page 80)

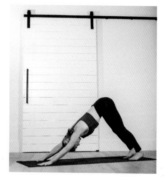

11 Repeat steps 5 through 10 on the left side and again one more time on each side. End in downward-facing dog (page 80) after your second time through on your left side.

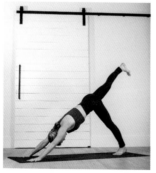

12 Inhale: down dog splits
(page 81)

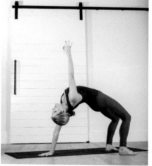

13 Flip dog for 5 breaths
(page 184)

> continued

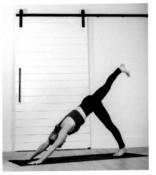

14 Inhale: down dog splits
(page 81)

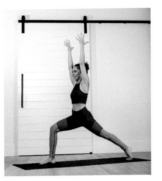

15 Crescent lunge for 5 breaths
(page 124)

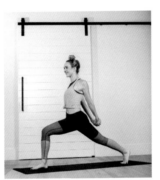

16 Crescent lunge with a
bind for 5 breaths
(page 125)

17 Vinyasa (page 98): repeat steps 12 through 16 on the other side.

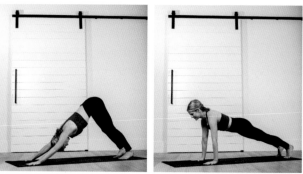

18 Once through the sequence on both sides, return to downward-facing dog, shift forward to high plank, and lower your body to the mat.

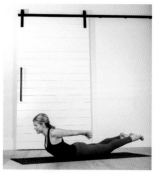

19 Locust with a bind for 2 rounds of 5 breaths each
(page 176)

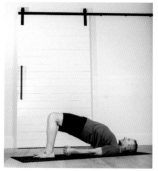

20 Bridge with a bind for 2 rounds of 5 breaths each
(page 181)

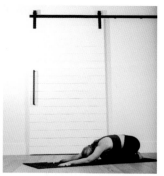

21 Child's pose for 5 breaths or more
(page 63)

15-Minute Upper-Body Sequence

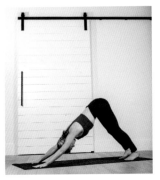

1 Downward-facing dog
for 5 breaths
(page 80)

2 Sun salutation A with cactus arms for 3 rounds
(page 107)

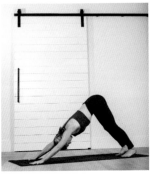

3 Downward-facing dog
for 5 breaths
(page 80)

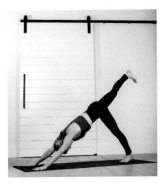

4 Down dog splits for
5 breaths
(page 81)

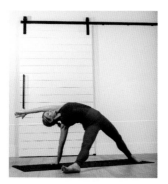

5 Fallen triangle for 5 breaths
(page 191)

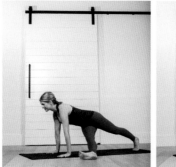 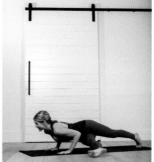

6 When you reground your lifted arm from fallen triangle, keep your legs extended as they are, bend your elbows, and lower to 90 degrees for a chaturanga variation.

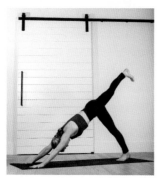 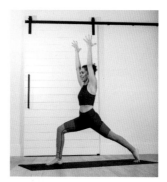

7 Down dog splits for 5 breaths
(page 81)

8 Crescent lunge for 5 breaths
(page 124)

> continued

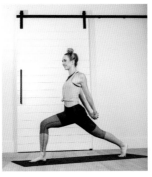

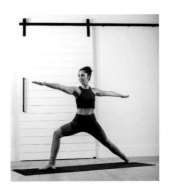

9 Crescent lunge with a
  bind for 5 breaths
  (page 125)

10 Warrior II for 5 breaths
   (page 117)

11 Vinyasa (page 98) for 5 breaths per pose on the first time through,
   except chaturanga. Repeat two more times at one breath per
   movement.

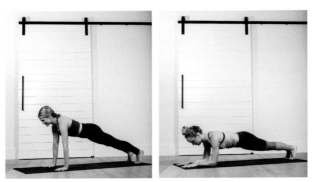

12 High plank to forearm plank for 5 rounds
   (pages 85 and 192)

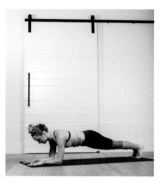

13 Forearm plank for 5 breaths
(page 192)

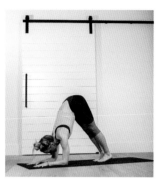

14 Dolphin for 5 breaths
(page 199)

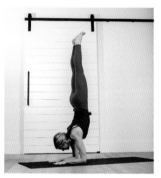

15 Forearm balance or
hops for 10 breaths
(page 200)

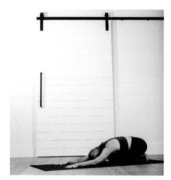

16 Child's pose for 5 breaths
or more
(page 63)

CHAPTER 10

Lower-Body Strength Sequences

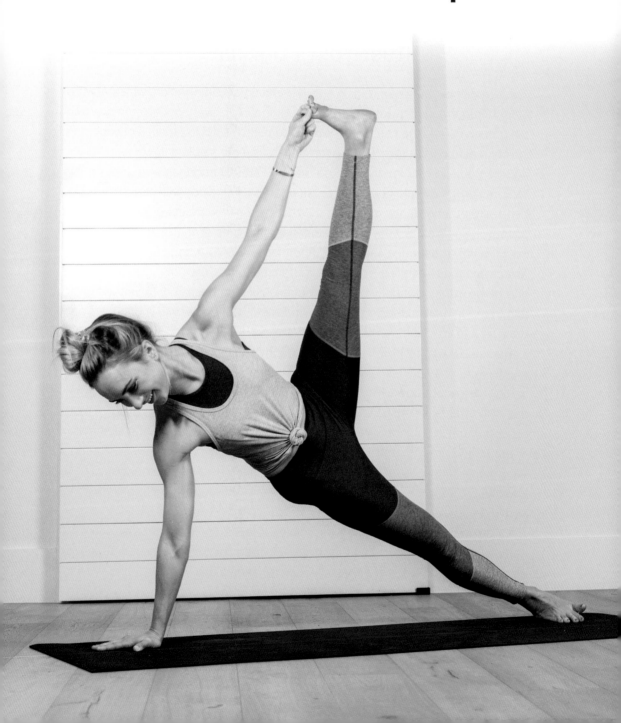

Strong legs and glutes do more than hold you up. They support your lower back, hips, and knees; stabilize your pelvis; free up your hip flexors; and support you in all areas of life. Because so many of us spend our days sitting in front of computers or in cars with our glutes and our leg muscles turned off, firing up these essential areas of the body takes some focus and effort. The sequences in this chapter are designed to strengthen and tone your butt and legs, boosting your power and confidence on and off the mat. These poses are physically challenging and require your focus and presence.

Trust Your Foundation

The strength of your pose begins with foundation and integration, which are created through rooting down, lifting, and hugging in. In every pose you move from the ground up and the center out. When you build a solid foundation of your pose in your feet and legs, your whole pose becomes more stable and centered. If you are not stable in your feet or your leg muscles are not engaged and drawing into your center, your whole pose can feel shaky. However, a tree with strong roots can bend, adapt, and dance in the wind. When you set your strong foundation in a pose, you can start to work the alignment and the lines of energy from the ground up, creating a shape that feels good and that serves your body and your energy. To activate the strength of your standing poses, press down firmly into your feet and harness the power of your large leg muscles. From the floor to your core, lift, and from your core to the floor, root down. Gather your power into your center, and draw up into your core.

Remember that all power principles are physical but are also connected to so much more—they are also energetic and spiritual. As you build strength, you start to move with more power, purpose, and trust. Strong legs and a firm footing off the mat helps you feel more balanced and centered. In power yoga, this boost of muscular strength is balanced with release. If you are just building muscular strength or are always striving for what's next, you miss the other side of power. Effort and ease create wholeness. As you activate, build, and tone the large muscles of your lower body, it's just as important to notice when and where you are overexerting and invite awareness and trust.

When you build a solid base—through your feet in the pose and through your committed practice—trust that the poses will open uniquely for you. The opening comes from being OK with all that you can do and all that you can't, and trusting the process. This is the spiritual shift that happens in yoga practice. You don't have to work so hard to control your experience within the pose. You can trust that as you embody your power, your pose and path forward will unfold. As you do the work, trust that everything else will work out. Clarity and calm come through your experience of your strength rather than how you think it should be.

In the yoga tradition, equanimity is the foundation of happiness and well-being. As you commit to your daily practice of power yoga, you will get stronger, and stress, imbalance, and tightness begin to fade, both physically and mentally. When your mind gets calm, you naturally start to feel more happy, centered, grateful, compassionate, and kind. These are the beautiful side effects of building strength and trust through a power yoga practice.

Lower-Body Sequences

The following poses and sequences will strengthen and tone your legs and butt, create stability in your body, and boost your confidence as you move on your yoga mat and walk through life. These poses demand your full presence, so set your drishti in each pose in order to stay present and tap into your full power.

Establish your foundation and build poses that utilize your powerful leg muscles. Press down into your feet, lift your power into your core, and hug into your centerline. With your strong foundation, you can start to work the lines of energy within your body and trust that the pose will open in a way that serves you.

You can practice these power-boosting sequences independently or work them into your practice to build more lower-body strength and stability.

5-Minute Lower-Body Sequence

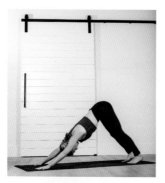

1 Downward-facing dog for 5 breaths
(page 80)

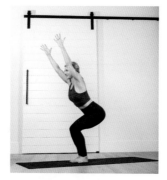

2 Chair pose for 5 breaths
(page 90)

> *continued*

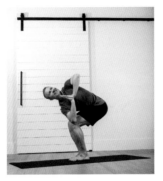

3 Chair twist for 5 breaths
  each side
  (page 153)

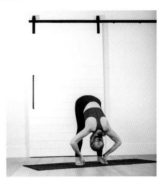

4 Big toe pose for 5 breaths
  (page 134)

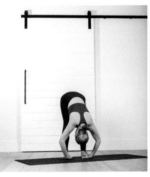

5 Gorilla for 5 breaths
  (page 135)

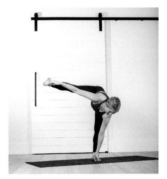

6 Big toe pose leg lifts for 5
  breaths at the top, repeating
  twice on each leg
  (page 134)

10-Minute Lower-Body Sequence

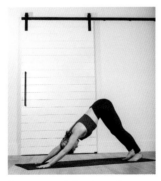

1 Downward-facing dog
  for 5 breaths
  (page 80)

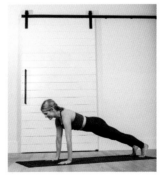

2 High plank for 5 breaths
  (page 85)

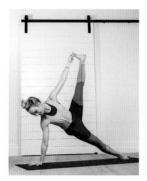
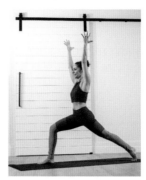
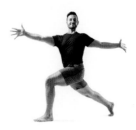

3 Full side plank
for 5 breaths
(page 190)

4 Crescent lunge
for 5 breaths
(page 124)

5 Open-arm crescent
twist
(page 156)

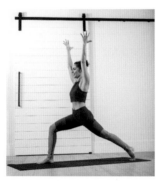
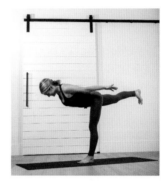

6 Crescent lunge
for 5 breaths
(page 124)

7 Airplane for 5 breaths
(page 150)

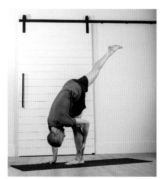
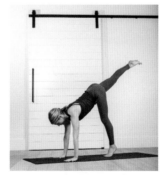

8 Standing splits
for 5 breaths
(page 151)

9 Handstand hops for 5
breaths (prep shown)
(page 203)

> continued

10 Vinyasa (page 98) and repeat on the other side. Move through the sequence one more time at one breath per movement.

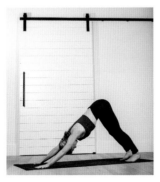

11 Downward-facing dog for 5 breaths
(page 80)

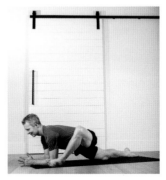

12 Lizard for 10 breaths
(page 232)

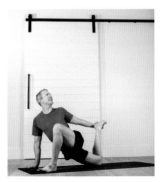

13 Lizard twist for 5 breaths
(page 232)

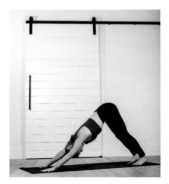

14 Downward-facing dog for 5 breaths
(page 80)

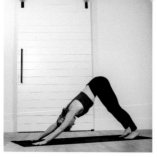

1 Downward-facing dog
for 5 breaths
(page 80)

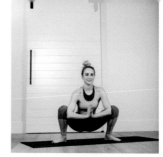

2 Jump forward into a yogi
squat for 5 breaths first time
through, then 1 breath after
(page 137)

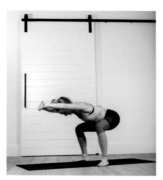

3 Bear pose for 5 breaths
(page 138)

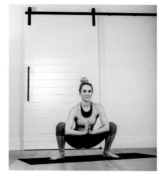

4 Yogi squat for 5 breaths
first time through, then
1 breath after
(page 137)

> continued

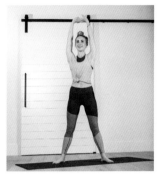

5 Mountain pose with
wide legs and fingers
interlaced for 1 breath
(page 77)

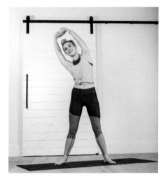

6 Mountain pose and
side bend to the right
for 1 breath
(page 77)

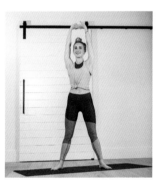

7 Mountain pose with
wide legs and fingers
interlaced for 1 breath
(page 77)

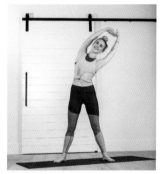

8 Mountain pose and
side bend to the left
for 1 breath
(page 77)

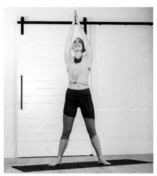

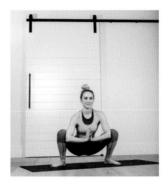

9 Mountain pose with palms united overhead for 1 breath
(page 77)

10 Yogi squat (page 137), then plant your hands on the ground.

11 Vinyasa (page 98) and repeat on the other side. Move through the sequence three times.

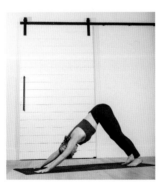

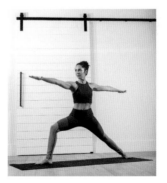

12 Downward-facing dog for 5 breaths
(page 80)

13 Warrior II for 5 breaths
(page 117)

> continued

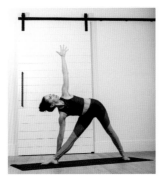

14 Triangle for 5 breaths
(page 121)

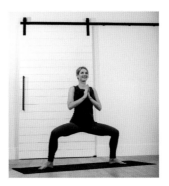

15 Goddess pose for 5 breaths
(page 132)

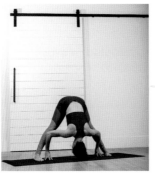

16 Wide-leg forward fold
for 5 breaths
(page 128)

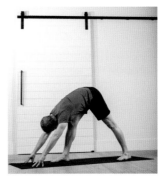

17 Pyramid pose for 5 breaths
(page 131)

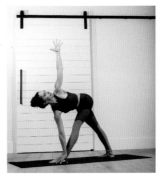

18 Twisting triangle for 5 breaths
(page 158)

19 Vinyasa (page 98) and switch sides. Then, repeat two more times at 1 breath per movement.

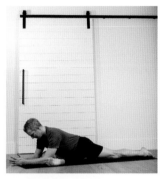

20 Half pigeon for 10 breaths each side
(page 224)

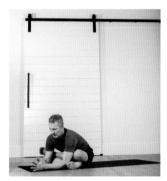

21 Double pigeon for 10 breaths each side
(page 226)

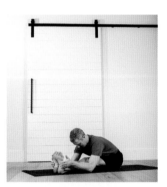

22 Seated forward fold for 10 breaths
(page 235)

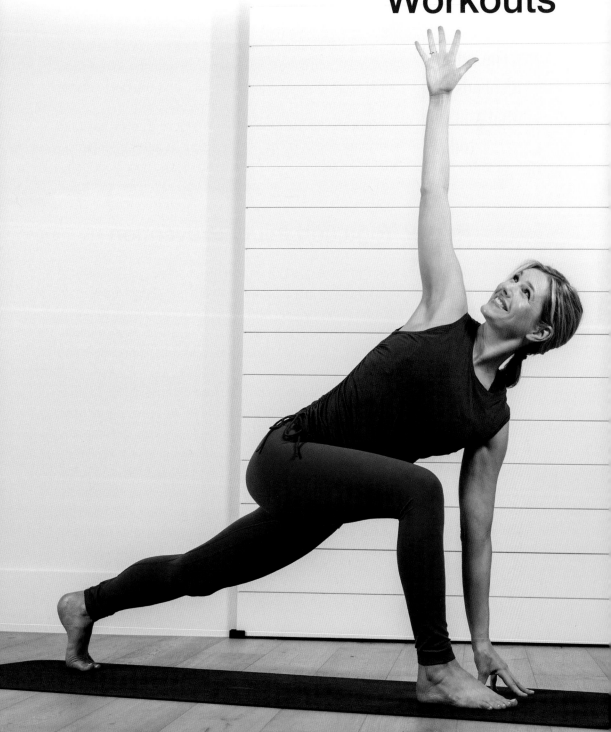

CHAPTER 11

Yoga Within Your Other Workouts

Power yoga is a natural complement to any athletic practice. Adding power yoga to your workouts and active lifestyle will provide cross-training to enhance your overall fitness, strengthen and tone all your major muscle groups, increase your flexibility, improve your posture, and build muscle memory to support you in other sports. Power yoga is a holistic workout that synthesizes mindfulness and movement, amplifying your results.

> The future depends on what you do today.
>
> Mahatma Gandhi

Your yoga practice is adaptable to meet your needs and doesn't need to look a certain way, which makes power yoga a great addition to any sport. Plus, you don't need any equipment, and there is no set time requirement. You can add power yoga to your current workouts, and you get to create your practice in the way that best serves you.

In this chapter, we'll look at how integrating power yoga into your other workouts can enhance your athletic performance, prevent injuries, increase your flexibility, and hone your focus. We'll also review some sport-specific sequences.

Power Yoga and Injury Prevention

In nature, like attracts like. The same goes for us as athletes. When you are used to a high-intensity workout, a challenging ride, or the rush of a fast-paced team sport, your body and mind crave the same intensity and stimulation. You get into a rhythm, and your sport becomes your lifestyle. But too much of anything creates imbalance over time, and in the body, this can easily lead to weakness, exhaustion, and injury.

You need to generate power for all sports, but you also need flexibility. There is an epidemic of injuries with serious athletes, especially when we are overly focused on being muscular and strong. Power yoga helps cultivate physical balance and develop the union between the effort of your sport and ease in your body. When you are used to pushing yourself to the limit, yoga can add much-needed restoration. As you pay attention to the feedback from your body, you will develop better body awareness and discover the right balance of stress and rest that works for you. Knowing your edges and learning when to pull back from overexertion, will help reduce your risk of injury and shorten your recovery time between workouts. Introducing new physical skills, working your body in different ways, and varying your training will help decrease your susceptibility to injury and improve overall athletic performance.

When you are training for a specific goal or competition, it's important to be mindful about how and when you integrate your yoga practice into your training schedule.

Power yoga is fantastic when you are building your physical and mental base during your precompetition period. For instance, if you are prepping for a CrossFit competition, power yoga would be an excellent addition during your initial training phase. As you get closer to the competition, you'll want to reduce the intensity of your yoga practice and shift your attention to building for your specific sport. When you are building your base of strength, power yoga will help amplify your power. The easier (or less intense) the sport-specific training you are doing, the more intense you want your yoga practice to be, and vice versa. During competition season, you don't want to stretch too much and compromise the integrity of your strength and structure. As you get closer to your peak, you'll want to focus more on recovery and clarity.

In power yoga, you use your body weight to tone and strengthen, which will work muscle groups that your main sport or activity typically won't engage. Yoga poses target specific areas of the body, but the poses also require a coordinated effort and total body integration. The combination of methodically flowing with breath and longer holds within poses will ignite your body and make your muscles burn in a whole new way. The combination of active and passive stretching combined with building strength creates ideal physical therapy for any sport.

If you are an athlete seeking specific results, power yoga will help you refine and focus your efforts to create new possibilities in your body. For instance, if you are a strength athlete looking for shoulder and hip flexibility, you can practice opening and recovery sequences to create more balanced action throughout your entire body. These sequences can be integrated into what you're already doing or can supplement your existing workout. If you are getting back into a routine at the gym and looking for more coordinated movement, you can do core sequences after your workouts to bring more targeted results that really matter to you. If you're an elite athlete with great proficiency in your body and movement, the emphasis of breath and intention in a meditative practice can help you achieve the mental edge you're looking for.

Sport-Specific Yoga Sequences

Your yoga practice will complement your training, support you in enhanced athletic performance, and prepare your body for your long-lasting practice of movement. There is no rush to the finish line or to a specific pose, so don't worry about getting

> Health is wealth.
> Peace of mind is
> happiness. Yoga
> shows the way.
>
> Swami Vishnudevananda

into extreme poses. It's about feeling good in your body and setting yourself up for the long game, so keep this in mind as you move on your mat.

When I found power yoga, it felt like a homecoming. I spent so much of my youth playing teams sports, and my body craved the consistent challenge and wisdom that comes through movement. On the flip side, I was still working on top of old injuries, scar tissue, and holding patterns that I'd developed early on, so I was breaking down. I couldn't generate the power I was used to and that I needed to stay consistent in sports as an adult. Power yoga helped me to unwind my tissues, open new energy, and embody my power in a completely new way.

Yoga is designed to bring the body, mind, and spirit together and to be an ongoing and lifelong practice. It's yoga, not just stretching. The results unfold over time, so be patient and stay committed. You don't make it to the finals by showing up for practice occasionally. Approach your power yoga practice with the same mindset and commitment. And, of course, have fun.

These sport-specific sequences can be practiced on their own, added to the end of your regular workout, or plugged into a longer power yoga practice. I suggest warming up for all these sequences with an opening pose, like child's pose, to get centered and generate your ujjayi breath. Once your focus is inward, continue your warm-up with a few rounds of sun salutation A's and B's. After you complete your sequence, take at least five minutes for a restorative final rest.

RESPECTING YOUR LIMITS

My rule of thumb is if it hurts, don't do it. The aim of yoga is to balance effort and ease, and the practice of yoga helps you distinguish the difference between discomfort and pain. It's essential to tune in to the communication from your body and to your edge. There's no glory in putting yourself in painful positions, whether it's in a yoga pose, work environment, or relationship. Pain creates suffering. However, being uncomfortable is part of growth. It's necessary to extend past your limits to increase your skills and effectiveness and create new results. In yoga, you'll build body awareness to understand your unique balance between too much and not enough and your sweet spot within every pose. Listen and honor your body, rather than pushing past your edge. When a yoga pose hurts, that's your body's signal to back off. Adjust your pose and build a shape that takes you to your edge and breathe into what you feel. Remember, you don't win at yoga; it's a process. Yoga teaches you how to compassionately respect the limitations of your body.

Running

Runners maximize power by using the strength of the whole body, not just strong legs. Running requires total body coordination and balance with each stride, and adding power poses to your workouts will illuminate areas that haven't been a focus in your runs. This sequence will help you both strengthen and open your hips, hamstrings, quads, glutes, and lower back.

Yoga is a fantastic cool-down after a run and offers release and rehab. The top comment I hear from my students who run is that yoga helps them to feel less sore. With yoga, you'll soothe your muscles, increase your flexibility, create more stability, and build more peace of mind. Once you get into your flow with yoga, you can tap into the same meditative quality that you cultivate on a great run.

1. Downward-Facing Dog (page 80)

Downward-facing dog distributes your power and builds whole body coordination as your root through both your hands and feet. It works on overall flexibility, decompresses the spine, and calms the nervous system. Down dog is a soothing stretch for the calves and hamstrings, and it can help prevent shin splints. This is a great pose to add before and after your runs. Place your hands shoulder-distance apart at the top of your mat and set your feet at the back of your mat.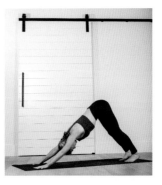
Lift your hips up into the air and create an inverted V shape. Separate your feet hip-width apart and keep your knees slightly bent as you pull your thigh bones back and press your heels toward the mat. Let your head hang down, and set your gaze between your ankles. Hold for 5 breaths. Use this pose as home base between poses. Check in to notice how your body responds to your different movements and stretches.

2. Low Crescent Lunge (page 125)

From downward-facing dog, step your right foot forward to your right thumb. Make sure your right knee is directly stacked over your ankle, even if that means using your hands to move your front foot forward. Set your left knee down on the mat and walk it back just a little to get into your psoas. Pull your legs toward one another and gather your power into your center. On your inhale, lift your chest and arms. Take a few deep breaths to fill your shape, and then press your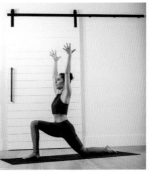

> continued

hips forward to access your psoas and hip flexors. Send your breath to these muscles that support your strides. Hold for 5 to 10 breaths, then step back to downward-facing dog and repeat on the other side.

3. Half Splits (page 229)

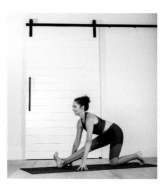

Half splits is often referred to as runner's lunge because of the specific benefits for tight legs. It is a deep stretch for the hamstrings and iliotibial band and will help soothe and open the large muscles of your powerful legs.

Come into a low lunge, with your right leg forward and your back knee on the ground. Tuck your back toes. Pull your hips back over your left knee, straighten your right leg, and flex your right foot. Pull the outer edge of your front foot back. As you activate your front foot, you'll target and soothe your iliotibial band. Drag your right hip crease back and down.

This is a great place to use blocks under your hands for support. Hold for 10 breaths, or more if you'd like. To come out of the pose, shift your weight forward onto your front foot, move through a low lunge, and make your way back to downward-facing dog. Repeat on the other side.

4. Fire Toes (page 136)

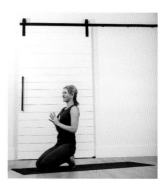

Fire toes will stretch and open all the muscles of your feet. This is a great pose to work in every day after your runs.

From downward-facing dog, drop down to your knees into a kneeling position. Tuck your toes under and sit back on your heels. Hug your inner ankles together, squeeze your legs toward your centerline, and lift your hands to prayer. Slide your tailbone down, engage your low belly, and breathe steadily as you continue to stoke your inner fire. Hold for 5 to 10 deep breaths. Think of all the good you are doing for your feet that support you on your long runs. To come out of the pose, place your palms on the ground, untuck your toes, and flap out your feet on your mat. Then press up to downward-facing dog.

5. Half Pigeon (page 224)

Half pigeon helps alleviate tension in a runner's strong and stable hips, lubricates the hip joints, and helps prevent injury. It's an effective stretch for the hip and piriformis muscle of the front leg and the psoas of the back leg, muscles that are usually tight in runners and athletes and hold tension from daily activities like sitting and driving.

From downward-facing dog, step your right knee toward your right wrist, your foot toward your left wrist, and lower yourself down onto your mat. The more parallel your shin is to the top of the mat, the deeper the pose, and you can pull your front heel closer to you to lessen the intensity. Extend your left leg behind you and point your toes to the back of your mat. Square both hips toward the ground. You can place your block under your right hip for more support. Reach your arms forward and fold your chest toward the ground into half pigeon. Rest your forehead on the ground or a block or prop yourself up on your forearms. Hold for 10 to 20 breaths. Walk your hands back under your shoulders and press back to downward-facing dog. Repeat on the left side.

6. Bound Angle (page 228)

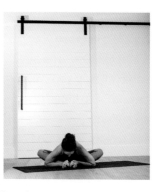

This pose is great for anyone who spends a lot of time sitting or walking, and it holds immense benefits for runners. Bound angle opens and lengthen the lower back, hips, and inner thighs. Be seated, bend your knees, and bring the soles of your feet together. Pull your heels close to your pelvis and hold the tops of your feet. Root down through your seat and sit up tall. With your exhale, keep hold of your feet and begin to hinge forward at your hips. Focus on lengthening your spine, even if that means not folding forward. This will help release your lower back, which takes much of the impact of your runs. Bend your elbows out to the sides. Use your arms to press on your legs to get lower to the ground and encourage a deeper opening of your hips. Let your head and neck release down. Hold for 10 breaths or more.

> continued

7. Legs-Up-the-Wall (page 207)

This pose is so good for the lower back. Legs-up-the-wall pose sets your thigh bones back and makes space in your lower back. This restorative inversion allows all your muscles to relax after a long run and for energy to flow from the ignited muscles of your legs back to your vital organs.

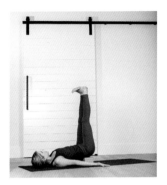

Sit on the floor with one hip bone against the wall. Lie on your back and lift your legs up the wall. Alternatively, you can place your block under your sacrum and lift your heels to the sky, as shown. Allow the weight of your legs to set your thigh bones back and expand your lower back. Extend your arms by your sides and turn your palms up to the sky as a symbol that you are open and ready to receive. Hold for 20 breaths or more. To come out of the pose, squeeze your knees into your chest, wiggle away from the wall or remove your block, gently roll over to one side, and make your way into a simple seat.

CrossFit

On the surface, yoga and CrossFit don't have a lot in common, which is why they're a great match. There is power in opposites. Yoga provides incredible cross-training for high-intensity workouts. Incorporating power yoga into your CrossFit regimen can help improve your flexibility, stability and range of motion and enhance recovery and relaxation. The static holds, dynamic stretches, and rhythmic breath in power yoga will help you cultivate a meditative awareness and excel in your workout of the day (WODs). Plus, power yoga will satisfy your desire for variation in your workouts and intensity, yielding serious results.

CrossFit and yoga create similar cultures, and the community, or sangha, is a huge part of both practices. When you build your foundation for your yoga with the practices in this book, you can show up with more confidence at your local yoga studio or CrossFit box. In both places, you'll connect with a tribe of people who are committed to a healthy lifestyle and who are moving and living with intention.

1. Easy Pose (page 70)

Sit with your ankles crossed. Lift through the crown of your head to lengthen your spine. If this is painful at all, you can either sit on a block to bring some relief to your hip flexors or place two blocks under your knees for support.

Once you feel comfortable, close your eyes and take a few deep breaths. Allow your energy to settle within you. Visualize chalk from your hands falling to the floor and allow the same to happen within you as you allow your energy to settle. Notice how you feel today. Notice the sensations within your body and what areas within you are calling for some attention and soothing.

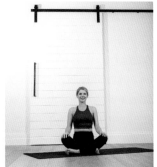

With your eyes still closed, set your intention for your practice. Take five more deep breaths here, with your mind aligning with how you want to feel and what you want to create in your yoga practice.

2. Downward-Facing Dog (page 80)

Downward-facing dog engages your full body and is an active stretch for two key areas for CrossFit athletes—the calf muscles and shoulders. As you press your thighs back and your heels down, you'll open and keep your calf muscles pliable. This is key as you lift and drive from your heels. As you press down through all four corners of your hands, you lengthen the side of your body and allow the neck and shoulders to unwind. Hold for 5 to 10 breaths.

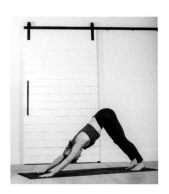

3. Standing Forward Fold With a Bind (page 83)

Standing forward fold helps unwind the muscles along the spine and neck, and adding the bind will open your shoulders, chest, and back. Don't worry if you can't reach your hands in your fold; this is a great place to use your strap, towel, or even your shirt as a connector. From downward-facing dog, walk your hands to the back of your mat and come into a standing forward fold. Start with your fingertips on the ground for support, take a few deep breaths, and let your neck relax

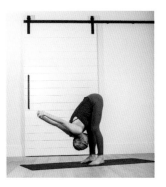

toward the ground. Then bring your focus to your feet, press down, and engage your leg muscles. With your firm base established, add the bind of your arms. Bend your elbows deeply, interlace your fingers at your lower back, and start to straighten your arms. It may feel good to bend your knees even more once you have the bind.

Hold for 5 to 10 breaths. Release your hands back to the mat and walk your hands forward into downward-facing dog.

> continued

4. Warrior I (page 91)

Warrior I builds total body integration and focus as well as ankle stability, which is crucial in squats and injury prevention. In your wide warrior stance, pay close attention to the alignment of your feet and legs to build ankle strength. Root down through all four corners of both feet and lift through your arches. Seal the pinkie toe edge of your back foot on your mat. As you press down through your back heel, engage your back leg fully and steer that hip bone forward. Look down at

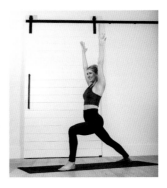

your front foot and ensure that you can see your big toe. The front knee tends to collapse in. Bring your front knee toward the outer edge of your foot, press down through your big toe mound and your heel, and scrub your heel toward the back of your mat. This will activate your hamstring and strengthen your quad.

Hold for 5 to 10 breaths, then step back to downward-facing dog or take a vinyasa. Repeat on the other side.

5. Bridge (page 180)

This front-body opener will help relieve the hip flexors and counteract bringing your knees toward your chest as you do in squats, burpees, box jumps, and so much more.

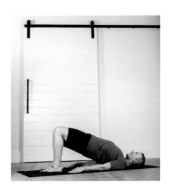

Lie on your back, separate your feet to hip-width apart, and walk your heels right under your knees. Press down with your feet and engage your legs and your core to lift your hips up. Lengthen your tailbone toward your knees and extend your chest toward your chin. Hold for 5 to 10 deep breaths. Repeat twice.

6. Lizard (page 232)

Lizard is a deep lunge that targets and opens the hip flexors and psoas. These muscles tighten from running, squatting, and jumping.

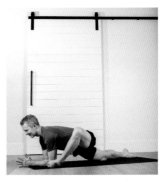

From downward-facing dog, bring your thumbs to touch at the top of your mat. Step your right foot to your right pinkie finger and turn your toes out to two o'clock. Press into your hands. Take a big breath in and lengthen your chest forward. Place your left knee down and walk it back slightly to go onto the front of your knee to open your hip flexor. You can stay here, or you can work down to your forearms on blocks or to your mat. Relax your head and your neck, and soften your chest toward the ground. Hold for 10 deep breaths. Press back to down dog. Repeat on the other side (shown).

7. Supine Twist (page 69)

This twist is soothing for the lower back and helps you unwind compression from heavy lifts and running.

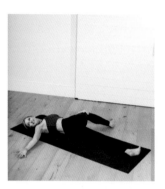

Lie on your back and squeeze both knees into your chest. Take a few deep breaths and rock side-to-side. Keep a hold of your right knee and extend your left leg long, with your heel on the mat. Cross your right knee to the left side of your mat for a twist. Take your arms out to a T. Hold for 10 breaths, then repeat on the other side.

Cycling

Cycling, like power yoga, is considered a low-impact activity and is grounded in breath. Cycling is a serious workout that builds incredible strength and endurance and gets your heart pumping. It can also create imbalance as cyclists often have very strong and overdeveloped quadriceps as well as tight hamstrings and hips. Being in the saddle, leaning forward toward your handlebars, with your spine constantly flexed forward, can take a serious toll on your posture. Power yoga helps cyclists address these physical imbalances by building optimal alignment, elongating tight and shortened muscles, cultivating core strength, and easing muscle pain and strain.

Your practice of drishti and rhythmic breath on the mat will help you stay focused while climbing and descending, and will improve your focus and calm your mind. When the ride starts to feel longer than it is, you'll be able to get into your groove, dig deeper, and unlock your inner strength. Your flexibility and focus will support you in every phase of your ride. And when you get back onto your mat, you'll use this inner power to stay steady in longer holds and find new possibilities in your poses.

> continued

1. Standing Forward Fold (page 83)

This standing forward fold unwinds the hamstrings, calves, and spine. It is an inversion with bent knees that helps restore the body and calm the nervous system as it circulates energy and oxygen to the brain. As you hang in your fold, allow the muscles of your neck, shoulders, and upper back that have been extended forward for hours in your ride to release. When you let go in your upper body, you'll open the flow of more oxygen-rich blood into your brain.

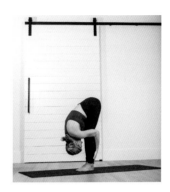

Stand with feet together and drape your torso over your thighs, hinging at your hips. You can widen your base and stand with feet hip-distance apart or wider for more support. Keep your knees bent to allow more of a stretch in your hamstrings and lower back. Either hold opposite elbows, catch your calves, or place your fingertips on the ground. Breathe into your upper back and hold for 10 breaths or more. Plant your hands to the ground and step back into downward-facing dog.

2. Reverse Warrior (page 118)

Reverse warrior utilizes the strength in your legs while also stretching your inner thighs, chest, lungs, and shoulders. As you lift your torso up and lean back to open the side of your body, you stretch the muscles between your ribs, the intercostals, which increases your breath capacity. From downward-facing dog, step your right foot forward, and rise to warrior II. Flip your front palm, reach your right hand up, and back toward the wall behind you, and reach your left arm

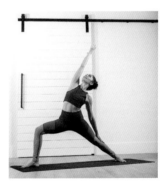

down your back leg. Peel open through the right side of your body and breathe into the spaces between your ribs. Lift and lengthen your front hip crease. Stay here for 5 breaths or more, and then return to warrior II. Stay on your right side and move into the next pose.

3. Humble Warrior (page 123)

In warrior II, interlace fingers at your lower back and create a bind. Bend your elbows, draw your shoulder blades together, and broaden across your chest. Straighten your arms and lift your chest as you breathe in. On your exhale, bow into humble warrior. Hug your right shoulder to the inside of your right knees and let your chest and head bow toward the earth. Stay strong through your legs and pull your right hip crease back. Lift your inhales into your upper back, and with each exhale, rinse away any tension in your shoulders. Set your drishti to your back ankle and hold for 5 breaths. On an inhale, rise to warrior II. Plant your hands to the top of the mat and either take a vinyasa or step back to downward-facing dog. Repeat reverse warrior and humble warrior on the left side.

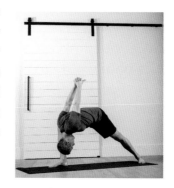

4. Low Lunge With a Quad Stretch (page 125)

Come into a low lunge with your right foot forward. Stack both hands on top of your right thigh. Hug your legs toward your centerline, lift your lower abdomen, and shift your hips more forward. Take a few deep breaths here to set your base and start to open the large muscles of your legs. When you feel steady and stable, bend your back knee and reach back with your left hand to catch your back foot for the quad stretch. You can use a strap or towel as a connector. Continue

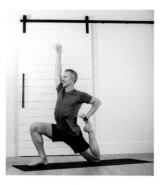

to root down through your front foot and pull your lower abdomen in and up. Lift your sternum, widen across your collar bones, and reach up with your right hand. Hold for 5 or more full rounds of breath. To come out of the pose, gently release your back foot, place both hands to the ground, and step back to downward-facing dog. Repeat on your second side.

5. Bridge With a Bind (page 181)

This front-body opener will help relieve the hip flexors and counteract bringing your knees toward your chest as you pedal for miles and miles. The addition of the arm bind will open your chest and release tension in your trapezius muscles. Lie on your back, separate your feet to hip-width distance, and walk your heels right under your knees. Press down with your feet and engage your legs and core to lift your hips up. Once you are lifted, interlace your fingers behind your back

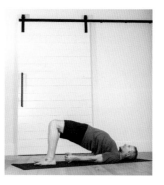

into a bind, and wiggle more onto your shoulder blades. Lengthen your tailbone toward your knees and extend your chest toward your chin. Hold for 5 to 10 deep breaths. Repeat twice.

> continued

6. Lizard Twist (page 232)

Lizard pose will help ease the tightness of your hip flexors and hamstrings, and the twist gives some extra juice for the quadriceps and opening across the chest.

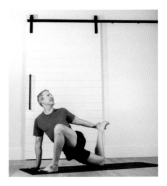

From downward-facing dog, bring the tips of your thumbs together. Step your right foot to the outside of your right pinkie finger and lower your back knee down. Turn your right toes out to two o'clock, shift to the outer edge of your foot, and allow your right hip to open. Stay lifted on your hands and reach your right arm to the back of the room and open across your chest. Bend your left knee and hold your left foot with your right hand. Pull your heel toward you and stretch your quadriceps. Squeeze your shoulder blades together and twist your chest up. Hold for 5 to 10 breaths. Release your left leg slowly and repeat on the other side (shown).

7. Cow Face Pose (page 227)

This pose gets deep into your hips, which never get to rest on your rides. It also stretches ankles, thighs, and lower back. Sit at the top of your mat, extend your left leg long, cross your right foot to the outside of your left thigh, and point your right knee to the sky. This may be enough of a stretch. To add on, slide your left heel back by your right hip. Stack your knees as much as possible, and adjust your feet by moving them closer to your body or away from you to find your sweet spot.

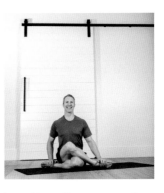

Press down through your seat, lift the crown of your head, and lengthen your spine. On your exhale, hinge at your hips and fold forward. Hold for 10 to 20 breaths. Slowly return to a seated position, unwind, and switch sides.

Team Sports

If you're training and getting hyped for your recreational sports leagues, power yoga will help you generate the strength, flexibility, and total body conditioning required to stay competitive. Power yoga will help you sharpen your skills for team sports that require a lot of running, cutting, jumping, and sprinting.

This sequence will help you build awareness of your whole body, improve your strength, increase your mobility, and propel you to new heights in your game. Balancing poses will build strength in your ankles and legs to empower explosive movements and increase your agility. Your drishti and breath will help hone your

Power yoga builds your focus and concentrated intention. Visually finding a focal point literally helps you keep your eye on the ball. In challenging asanas, your drishti helps you stay focused on your goal, and you develop concentration as you keep your mind on your breath. This is the mind-body connection.

Practicing pranayama, or breath control, in your power practice will help increase your endurance, enhance lung capacity, and focus your mind. You can use the simple technique of focusing on your breath before and after any practice or game to quickly return to your center.

In basketball, the goal is putting the ball through the hoop, and in running, the focus is getting to the finish line. In yoga, as you engage your whole body and move in coordination with your breath, your purposeful movements become a meditation in motion. This practice of mindfulness will sharpen your overall focus and automatically elevate your performance.

focus, and within the poses, you'll develop both power and grace that you can carry onto the field or court.

1. Dragonfly Twist (page 156)

This easy twist lengthens and opens your whole body and cultivates connection to your center. Start in downward-facing dog and step your right foot to your right thumb. Press onto your fingertips in this long lunge, and on your inhale, reach your chest forward. Lengthen your body from your back heel to your heart. On your next inhale, lift your right arm to the sky and rotate open along that line you just lengthened. Squeeze your front knee in toward your

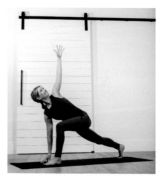

chest. The more your hug in, the more you can unwind and radiate out. Hold for 5 to 10 breaths, then step back to downward-facing dog and repeat on the other side (shown).

2. Warrior II (page 117)

Warrior II teaches us how to fill up space with purpose and power. It strengthens and stretches the quads, hamstrings, ankles, and hip flexors and sculpts the arms and back. From downward-facing dog, step your right foot to the top of your mat, spin your left heel down to the ground, and squeeze your heels toward one another to activate your legs. Once you've set your base, inhale to lift your chest and widen your arms. Your wrist should hover over your ankles. Expand

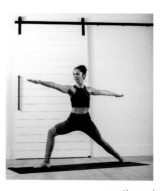

> continued

through your fingers and set your drishti over your front middle finger to hone your focus. Lift your breath up to your chest and fill your wingspan with energy. Hold for 5 to 10 breaths and either take a vinyasa or step back to downward-facing dog and repeat on the left side.

3. Triangle (page 121)

Triangle creates full-body expression as you press down, lift, and expand out in all directions. It increases the flexibility of hips and hamstrings, opens the chest, and creates a keen awareness of the core and center point of the body. From downward-facing dog, step your right foot forward and rise into warrior II. Straighten your front leg and reach your right arm and torso forward as long as you can. Plant your right fingers down to the earth or block and lift your left arm to the sky. Hold for 5 to 10 breaths. Vinyasa or step back to downward-facing dog. Repeat on the other side.

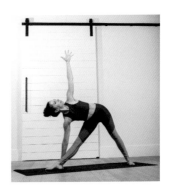

4. Tree (page 144)

Tree pose tones your legs, strengthens your core, and improves overall balance. As you stand on one foot, you will build stability in your feet and ankles. Remember that falling is part of the process and helps you find your center.

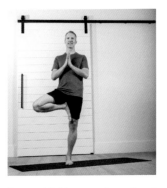

Step to the top of your mat and stand tall in mountain pose. Ground down through all four corners of your right foot and lift your left foot to the calf or inner thigh of your standing leg. Activate your core by pulling your belly button in and up and slide your tailbone down. Unite your hands at heart center or extend your arms like branches in a way that feels natural to you. Set your gaze to one point and hold for 10 deep breaths. Repeat on the other side (shown).

5. Dancer (page 146)

Dancer pose builds balance, coordination, and grace. The push and pull between the kick of your raised leg and the lift of your chest creates a dance between effort and ease, and in it, you discover your most powerful position. From mountain pose, anchor down into your right standing foot, bend your left knee, and catch your foot or ankle with your left hand.

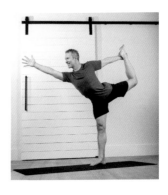

Extend your right arm to the sky. Pull your abdomen in to stabilize your center. Hug both knees toward your centerline. With an inhale, kick your lifted shin behind you and hold for 5 breaths. Return to standing to recenter and transition to the other side. Repeat twice on each side.

6. Floor Bow (page 177)

Bow pose is a dynamic backbend that opens your chest and shoulders, creates flexibility in your spine, and enhances your breath capacity. Lie on your stomach with your forehead on the mat. Bend your knees, grab your outer ankles or the tops of your feet, and pull your knees to hip-width apart. With your inhale, kick your shins back and lift your chest with the power from your legs. Allow your chest to open. Hold for 5 breaths and repeat twice. When you are complete with two rounds, press back into child's pose for a few recentering breaths.

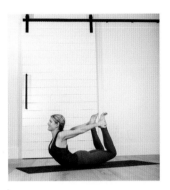

7. Single-Leg Forward Fold (page 236)

This pose stretches and release the calves, hamstrings, lower back, and shoulders. It's also calming for the mind and nervous system and gives you an opportunity to turn inward and focus on your breath. Be seated and extend your right leg. Bend your left knee, place your left foot against your inner right thigh, and create tree legs. Flex your right foot and firm your right leg muscles. You can bend your front leg as much as you need to; there are no extra points for straight

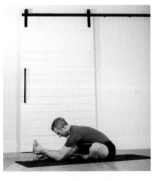

legs. On your inhale, sit up tall and reach your arms high. Exhale and hinge at your hips to fold forward. To take it deeper and target your quadratus lumborum muscle, cross your left hand to catch the outside edge of your right foot and pull your chest down and parallel to the mat. Hold for 10 to 20 breaths. Slowly return to a seated position, unwind your legs, and switch sides.

8. Seated Half Pigeon (page 225)

This seated pigeon variation releases the piriformis that is tight in almost all athletes. Once you open the hips, you'll unlock energy that's been held up in your tissues and free yourself up for greater mobility. Begin seated and place your hand behind your hips. Bend your knees, and plant your feet onto the ground. Sit up tall, lift your shoulders up by your ears, and roll your shoulders back to open across your

> continued

chest. The more you maintain the length of your spine and the broadness of your chest, the more space you create for your breath and energy to flow through you. Cross your right ankle over your left thigh and flex your foot. Move your left foot closer to you or further away to find the right amount of stretch for you. Hold for 10 breaths. Release your legs and switch sides.

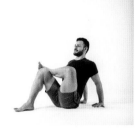

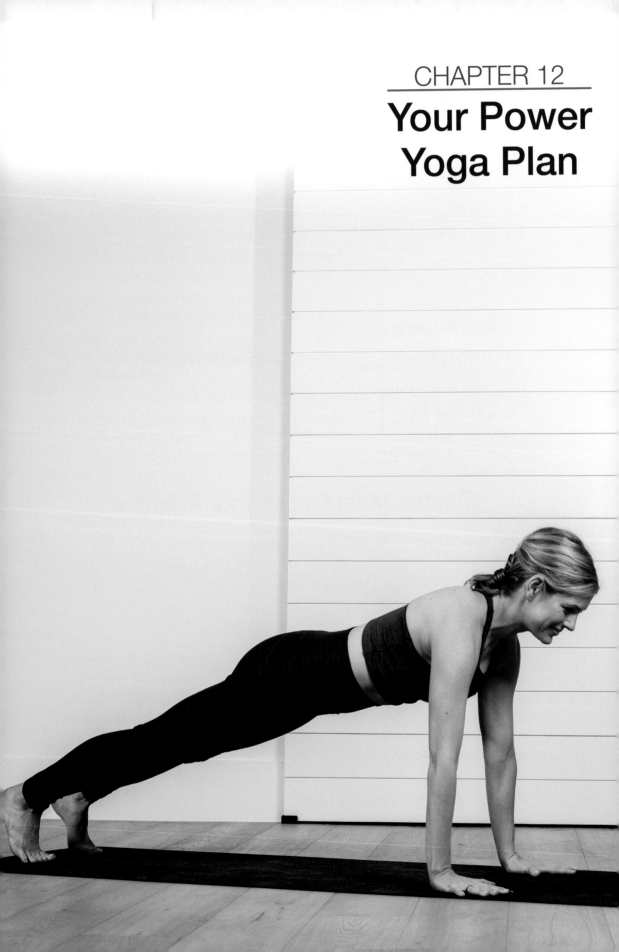

CHAPTER 12

Your Power Yoga Plan

Now it's time to get started. You have all the information and the tools that you need to begin your 28-day power yoga plan. This plan is accessible for anyone at any level because in power yoga, you determine what your plan looks like based on your needs, goals, and the results you want to create. Each week builds on the physical and mental benefits from the previous week. I'll provide you with a master sequence each week that you can do every day for the whole week. Trust that you'll have a holistic practice every day that will awaken and activate your body and breath.

> Realize deeply that the present moment is all you will ever have.
>
> Eckhart Tolle

If you are looking to create specific results in your practice, or if you want to change things up daily, you can also use the sequences outlined in the earlier chapters to build a plan that works for you. This gives you the freedom to customize your practice depending on how you feel and what your needs are that day, and it allows you to work with the intuition and inner wisdom that you will unlock as you grow your yoga practice. I also provide examples for building a custom flow each week and integrating the building blocks of a power yoga practice.

Get the Most Out of Your Practice

When you show up on your mat and practice every day for the next 28 days, you will transform your body, mind, and spirit. Here are a few tips and tools that I recommend to help you maximize your results.

Set Your Intention

Take time to set your intention and establish your energetic aim before each practice. Each time you get lost or distracted, use your intention as a reminder to realign with why you came to you mat. Pause between poses with your hands at your heart center and return to your intention and your breath. Yoga is skillfulness in action, and the more you infuse purpose into your poses, the more powerful your practice will be for you.

Focus on What You *Can* Do

We all ask ourselves questions like, "Why isn't my body doing this?" or "What is the teacher talking about?" or "How is that person doing that?" When this starts to happen, pause. Give thanks for what *is* happening in this moment and how your body is working for you in this pose. Honor your efforts and acknowledge yourself for what you can do. The more you practice, the easier it gets.

Stay in the Now

When your mind starts to take over and tries to take you out of the game, return to your breath. Use your breath to stay in the physical practice and in your body. When you are aware and connected to your breath, you are automatically in the now moment, which is the only place you have power. Yoga reminds us that *right now* is when life happens. When you are present and not worried about what's next, you get to choose to be purposeful, joyful, and relaxed with what's happening right now. Presence gives you power.

Celebrate Your Growth

What we celebrate, we expand. When you acknowledge and appreciate your growth, you invite more of the same, and your practice is fertile ground to practice gratitude. When new sensations arise, give thanks for the growth, the learning, and the process. One of the coolest things about this practice is that there is no end to yoga. Learning can look different every time you step on your mat.

Make Adaptations

Remember, everything is adaptable. Our bodies are different every day, and it's essential to work with how you are feeling to build a practice that best serves you. If you are feeling low energy and need a little boost, add more sun salutations and power poses into your practice. If you have excess energy from your day and want to wind down, you can practice a longer closing sequence focused on hips and forward folds. On days when you're feeling more introspective, you can use your practice to open and expand your energy and prepare you to go out and conquer your day. To challenge yourself or shift your energy, you can go upside down and practice inversions. If a shape feels good to you, linger there. If a pose doesn't work for you within a sequence, leave it out. Everything is adaptable.

> You must learn a new way to think before you can master a new way to be.
>
> Marianne Williamson

Trust the Practice

Yoga is a journey, not a destination. It's meant to be an ongoing practice that unfolds over time and is designed to be a lifelong practice. As you trust the inherent wisdom of this ancient practice and stay committed to your personal practice, the gifts of yoga are revealed to you.

TEACHING TIP

Your Class Outline

Every power yoga class will follow the same general blueprint of poses, intentions, and qualities. As a teacher, you can use this outline to set up and build your power yoga classes to create strong and empowering sequences. The progression from the opening through the cool-down will ensure that you deliver a holistic journey through the body and will free you to share authentically and inspire as you lead challenging, sweaty power yoga classes. As a practitioner, this outline will help you to create complete practices and discover what feels best for you.

Sequence	Poses	Intention	Qualities
Opening	Opening pose	Awaken the breath and body	Earth element, foundation, turning attention inward, shift from thinking to feeling, and establish rhythmic breath
Warm-up	Sun salutations	Link the breath with movement; get the whole body moving	Water element, utilize the whole body, ritual, and build inner heat
Power	Standing, balancing, and twists; power sequences	Build strength and endurance; find the edge and ease in every pose	Fire element, dynamic movement, building strength, focus, creative sequencing, and the deeply physical center of every power class
Peak	Backbends, arm balances, and inversions	More advanced poses and challenging holds	Air element, focus, skill, flexibility, expansion, precision, and apex of practice
Cool-down	Hips, folds, and final rest	Counterposes to a strengthening practice, longer holds, calm the nervous system	Space element, finishing poses, stretch, recover, acceptance, let go, surrender, and rest

Your Power Yoga Plan: Sequences

There are two ways that you can use the practices in this book to support you in all four weeks of your power yoga plan. I've outlined a master sequence for each week. Each practice emphasizes one of the principles of power and is designed to give you a holistic practice and deliver an embodied understanding of the foundational power yoga principles. You can use these sequences every day for four weeks as you build your practice.

The other option is to design your own practice using the sequences outlined in the previous chapters. If you want to create specific results, like upper-body strengthening, working up to handstand, or cultivating core strength, this approach helps you build a specific plan that works for you. This option gives you the freedom to change some or all of your practice, depending on your needs, goals, and how you feel. I've provided a blueprint and examples each week of "build your own" sequences that integrate all the elements of a well-rounded power yoga practice.

Whether you build your own sequences or use the master sequences outlined in this book, you will start with a 20-minute practice each day for the first week and gradually move up to 60-minutes of practice per day in your final week of the program. After 28 days of power yoga, you'll have built the physical strength and the mental focus to see real results in your body and in your life. As you engage your whole body with these power yoga foundational flows, you will not only enhance your athleticism but also prepare yourself to advance your yoga practice and go deeper—body, mind, and spirit.

For these 28 days, fully commit to your practice. Don't skip a practice because you don't have time. Simple shifts in your schedule will create big results in your body and energy. Even if it means breaking up your practice and weaving it in throughout your day, stick with your plan for these four weeks. It's better to do a little bit each day than to skip a day or double up another day. Get onto your mat daily, and I promise you'll feel the difference. Consistency is queen in creating results.

> The secret of change is to focus all your energy not on fighting the old but on building the new.
>
> Socrates

Week 1: Foundation

The key to building your power yoga practice is creating a solid foundation. You must stabilize before you mobilize. In every pose, work from the ground up and your center out to enhance your power yoga practice. As you create your strong foundation with your daily 20-minute practice in week one, you will start to build your strength and boost your overall power in your practice. As you feel stronger and more stable on the mat, you can start to tap into these strengths off the mat.

20-Minute Master Sequence

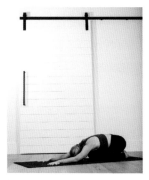

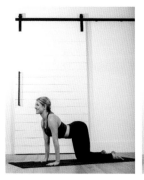

1 Child's pose for 20 breaths
(page 63)

2 Cat and cow for 5 breaths
(page 66)

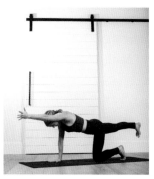

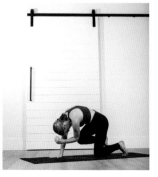

3 Extended tabletop on right side for 5 breaths
(page 65)

4 Tabletop crunches on right side for 5 breaths
(page 65)

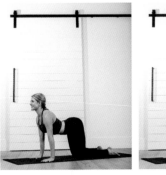

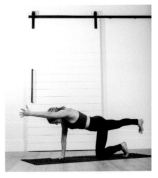

5 Cat and cow for 5 breaths
(page 66)

6 Extended tabletop on
left side for 5 breaths
(page 65)

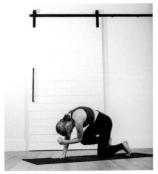

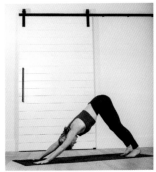

7 Tabletop crunches on left
side for 5 breaths
(page 65)

8 Downward-facing dog
for 5 breaths
(page 80)

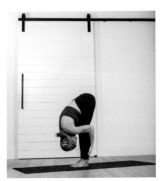

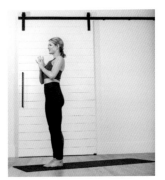

9 Standing forward fold
for 5 breaths
(page 83)

10 Mountain pose for an extended
breath, then bring hands to
heart for 3 breaths with Om
(page 77)

> continued

11 Sun salutation A for 3 rounds
(page 100)

12 Sun salutation B for 1 round (hold warrior 1 for 5 breaths)
(page 103)

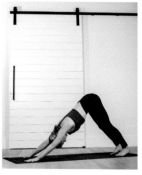 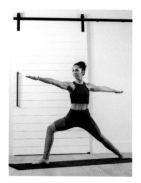 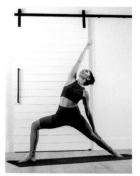

13 Downward-facing dog
for 5 breaths
(page 80)

14 Warrior II for 5 breaths
(page 117)

15 Reverse warrior
for 5 breaths
(page 118)

16 Vinyasa (page 98): repeat steps 13 to 16 on your left side.

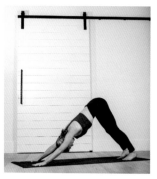 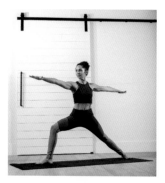

17 Downward-facing
dog for 5 breaths
(page 80)

18 Warrior II for 1 breath
(page 117)

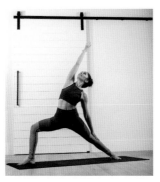

19 Reverse warrior for 1 breath
(page 118)

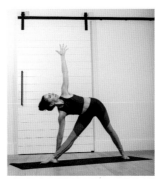

20 Triangle for 5 breaths
(page 121)

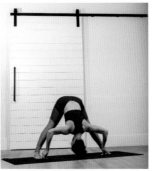

21 Wide-leg forward fold
for 5 breaths
(page 128)

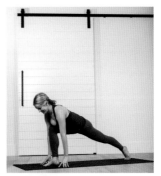

22 Low lunge for 1 breath
as a transition
(page 125)

23 Vinyasa (page 98). Repeat steps 17-23 on left side.

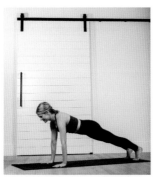

24 High plank for 5 breaths
(page 85)

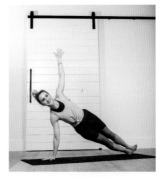

25 Side plank on right
side for 5 breaths
(page 190)

> *continued*

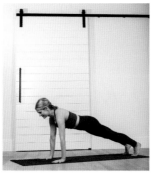

26 High plank for 5 breaths
(page 85)

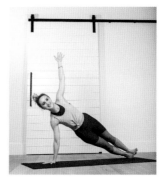

27 Side plank on left side
for 5 breaths
(page 190)

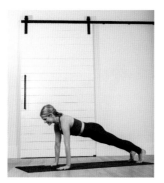

28 High plank for 5 breaths
(page 85)

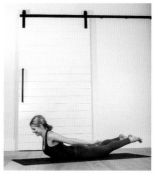

29 Lower to your mat into locust
for 2 rounds of 5 breaths each
(page 176)

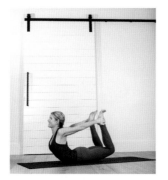

30 Floor bow for 2 rounds
of 5 breaths each
(page 177)

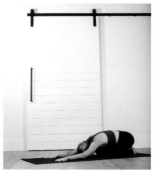

31 Child's pose for 5 breaths
(page 63)

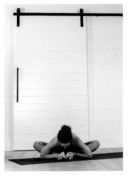

32 Bound angle
for 10 breaths
(page 228)

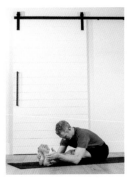

33 Seated forward fold
for 10 breaths
(page 235)

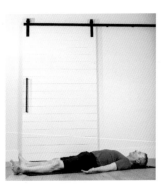

34 Final rest for 3 minutes
or more
(page 241)

Week 2: Focus

Practice this 30-minute sequence of focus-enhancing poses every day this week and build proficiency in finding your drishti from the start to finish of your practice. Allow your physical gaze to be the starting point of your stability. In every pose, draw your energy up and in. Pay attention to how your whole body moves and works as one powerful unit. Harness your focus and expand your physical power, and then bring this new level of precision to all that you do, on and off the mat. Remember, it's not about doing everything perfectly; it's about gracefully recovering when you lose focus.

30-Minute Master Sequence

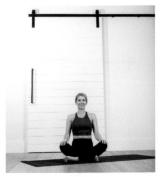

1 Easy pose for 10 breaths
(page 70)

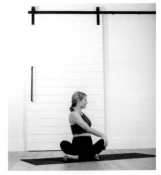

2 Easy seated twist for 5 breaths
each side; extend arms
overhead on an inhale to
center
(page 71)

> continued

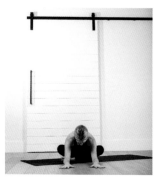

3 Easy seated fold
for 5 breaths
(page 71)

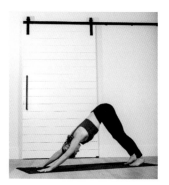

4 Downward-facing dog
for 5 breaths
(page 80)

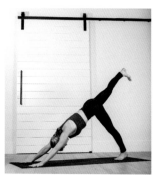

5 Down dog splits on
right side for 1 breath
(page 81)

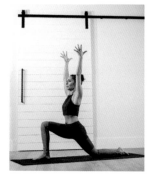

6 Low crescent lunge on
right side for 5 breaths
(page 125)

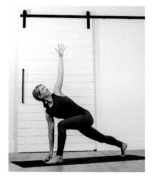

7 Dragonfly twist on right
side for 5 breaths
(page 156)

8 Repeat steps 4 to 7 on the left side.

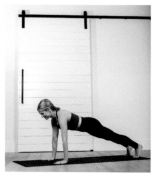

9 High plank for 5 breaths
(page 85)

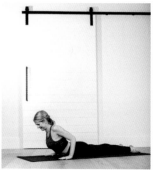

10 Lower to the mat into cobra
3 times with breath (inhale
lift; exhale lower)
(page 89)

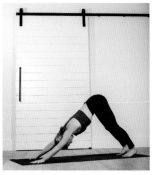

11 Downward-facing dog
for 5 breaths
(page 80)

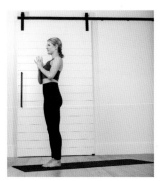

12 Mountain pose with upward
salute for 1 breath; then bring
hands to heart for 3 Oms
(page 77)

13 Sun salutation A: cactus arms variation (page 107) for 3 rounds.

14 Sun salutation B: chair twist variation (page 109) for 3 rounds.

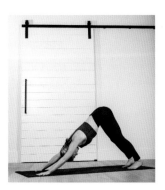

15 Downward-facing dog
for 5 breaths
(page 80)

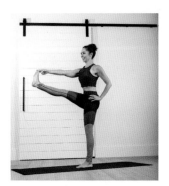

16 Standing leg raise on
right side for 5 breaths
(page 142)

> continued

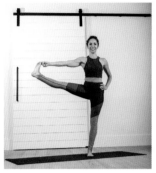

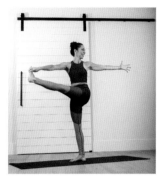

17 Standing side leg raise on right side for 5 breaths
(page 143)

18 Standing leg raise twist on right side for 5 breaths
(page 143)

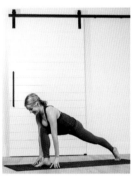

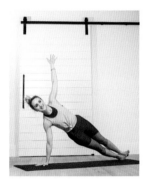

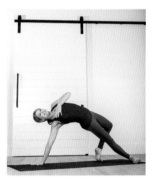

19 Low lunge on right side with both hands to the ground for 1 breath as a transition
(page 125)

20 Side plank on right side with left arm high for 5 breaths
(page 190)

21 Wild thing on right side for 5 breaths
(page 191)

22 Vinyasa (page 98). Repeat steps 15 to 21 on your left side.

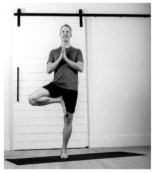

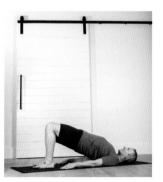

23 Tree pose for 10 breaths each side
(page 144)

24 Bridge for two rounds of 5 breaths each
(page 180)

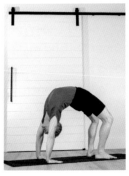

25 Wheel for two rounds
of 5 breaths
(page 182)

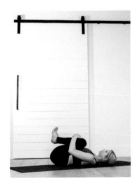

26 Knees-to-chest
(page 73)

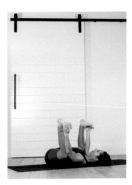

27 Happy baby
(page 231)

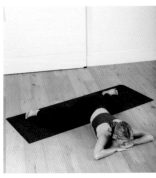

28 Frog for 20 breaths
(page 223)

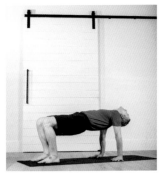

29 Reverse tabletop
for 5 breaths
(page 233)

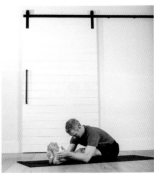

30 Seated forward fold
for 5 breaths
(page 235)

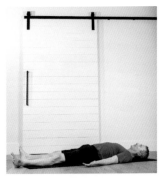

31 Final rest for 4 minutes
or more
(page 241)

Week 3: Fire

This foundational sequence will spark your inner power as you awaken your whole body. In this 45-minute core-centered sequence, we'll focus on heat-building poses, such as standing poses and twists, which will stoke your inner fire and make you feel alive. Heat melts away layers of resistance and old holding patterns, physically and energetically. Work your entire body to clear out the old, gain new energy, and burn brighter.

45-Minute Master Sequence

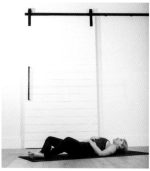
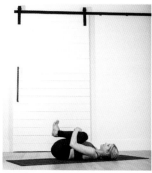

1   Reclined bound angle
    for 20 breaths
    (page 68)

2   Knees-to-chest
    for 5 breaths
    (page 73)

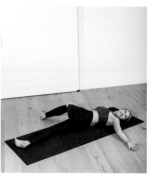
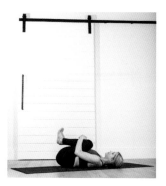

3   Supine twist for 5 breaths
    each side
    (page 69)

4   Knees-to-chest for 1 breath
    (page 73)

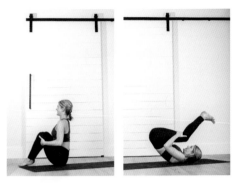

5 Rock 'n' rolls 5 times
(page 74)

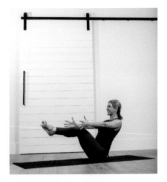

6 Boat for 5 breaths
(page 248)

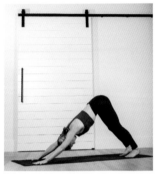

7 Downward-facing dog
for 5 breaths
(page 80)

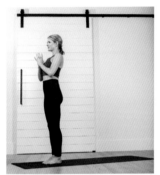

8 Mountain pose with upward
salute for 1 breath; then bring
hands to heart for 3 Oms
(page 77)

9 Sun salutation A: open-arm twist variation (page 106) for 3 rounds.

10 Sun salutation B: plank curls variation (page 112) for 3 rounds on each side.

> continued

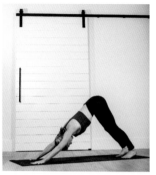

11 Downward-facing dog for 5 breaths
(page 80)

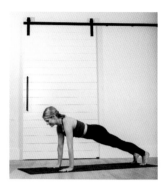

12 High plank for 5 breaths
(page 85)

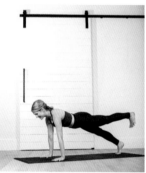

13 Three-point plank with right leg lifted for 5 breaths
(page 86)

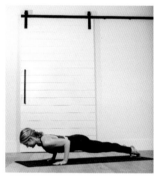

14 Exhale: low plank
(page 87)

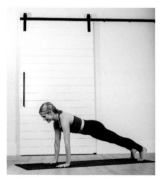

15 Inhale: high plank
(page 85)

16 Repeat steps 11 to 15 on your left side.

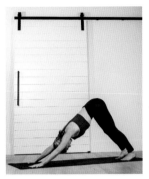

17 Downward-facing dog for 5 breaths
(page 80)

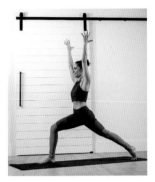

18 Crescent lunge on right side for 5 breaths
(page 124)

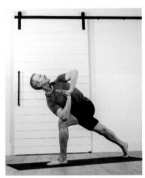

19 Crescent twist right side for 5 breaths
(page 155)

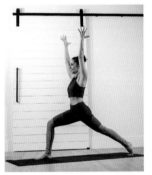

20 Crescent lunge on right side for 5 breaths
(page 124)

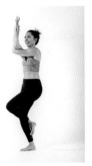

21 Eagle on right side for 5 breaths
(page 140)

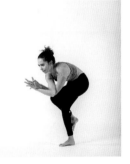

22 Nested eagle on right side for 5 breaths
(page 141)

> *continued*

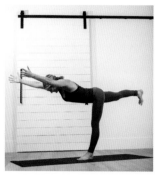

23 Warrior III on right side
for 5 breaths
(page 150)

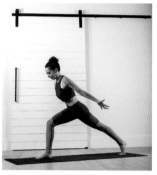

24 Lightning lunge on right side
with arms reaching back for
5 breaths
(page 126)

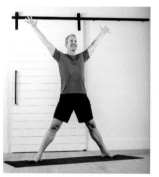

25 Star pose for 5 breaths
(page 127)

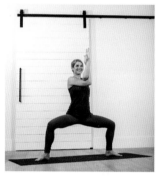

26 Goddess with eagle arms
(right arm under) for
5 breaths
(page 133)

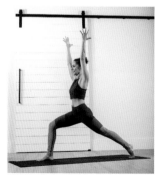

27 Crescent lunge on right
side for 5 breaths
(page 124)

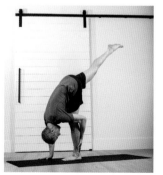

28 Standing splits on right
side for 5 breaths
(page 151)

29 Vinyasa (page 98). Repeat steps 27 to 39 on the left side; then repeat steps 27 to 39 one more time on each side at one breath per movement (except for downward-facing dog, which remains 5 breaths).

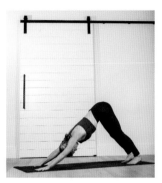

30 Downward-facing dog for 5 breaths
(page 80)

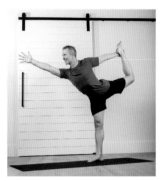

31 Dancer for two rounds of 5 breaths each side
(page 146)

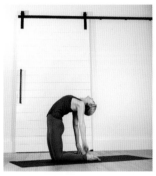

32 Camel for 2 rounds of 5 breaths; kneel or do hero pose between rounds
(page 179)

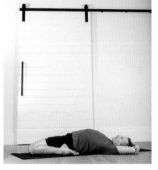

33 Reclined hero pose for 10 breaths
(page 178)

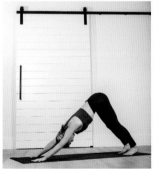

34 Downward-facing dog for 5 breaths
(page 80)

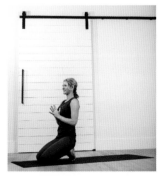

35 Fire toes pose for 10 breaths
(page 136)

> continued

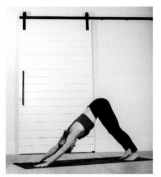

36 Downward-facing dog
for 5 breaths
(page 80)

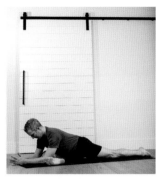

37 Half pigeon on right side
for 20 breaths
(page 224)

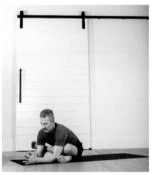

38 Double pigeon with left
leg on top for 20 breaths
(page 226)

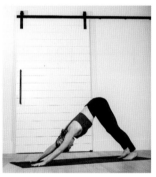

39 Downward-facing dog
for 5 breaths
(page 80)

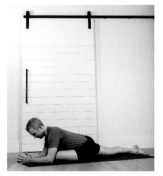

40 Half pigeon on left side
for 20 breaths
(page 224)

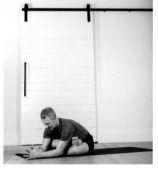

41 Double pigeon with right
leg on top for 20 breaths
(page 226)

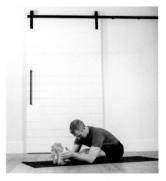

42 Seated forward fold
for 20 breaths
(page 235)

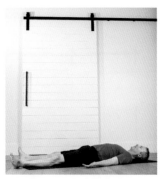

43 Final rest for 4 minutes
or more
(page 241)

Week 4: Flow

Keep your energetic river flowing in this dynamic 60-minute sequence that explores one breath with one movement. Bring fluidity into your powerful practice as you link your body and breath and allow this synchronization become a meditation in motion. When you surrender mental energy over to the physical practice, resistance fades and your energy surges. Fully commit to your breath and the present moment and flow like water from one pose to the next.

60-Minute Master Sequence

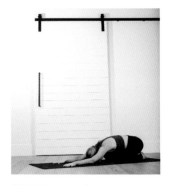

1 Child's pose for
20 breaths
(page 63)

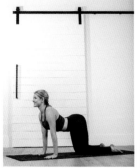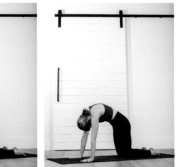

2 Cat and cow for 5 breaths
(page 66)

> continued

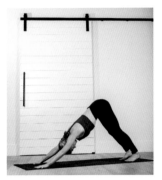

3 Downward-facing
dog for 5 breaths
(page 80)

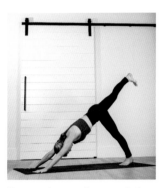

4 Down dog splits on right
side for 1 breath
(page 81)

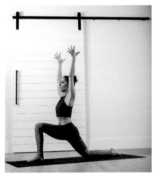

5 Low crescent lunge on
right side for 5 breaths
(page 125)

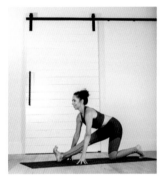

6 Half splits on right side
for 5 breaths
(page 229)

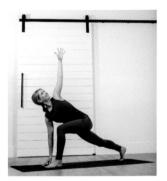

7 Dragonfly twist on right
side for 5 breaths
(page 156)

8 Repeat steps 3 to 7 on the left side.

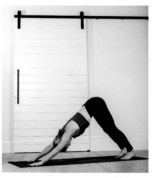

9 Downward-facing dog
for 5 breaths
(page 80)

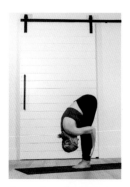

10 Standing forward
fold for 10 breaths
(page 83)

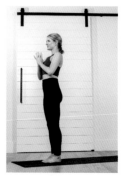

11 Mountain pose with
upward salute
for 1 breath; then
bring hands to
heart for 3 Oms
(page 78)

12 Sun salutation A: side bend variation (page 108) for 5 rounds.

13 Sun salutation B: open-arm chair twist variation (page 154) for 4 rounds
(hold twists and warrior 1 for 5 breaths the first time through, then 1
breath per movement for next three rounds).

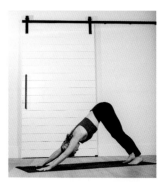

14 Downward-facing dog
for 5 breaths
(page 80)

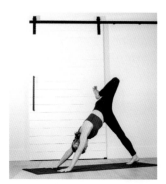

15 Down dog splits on right side,
with bent knee for 5 breaths
(page 81)

> continued

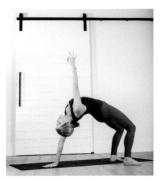

16 Flip dog to the right for 5 breaths
(page 184)

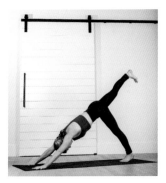

17 Down dog splits on right side for 1 breath
(page 81)

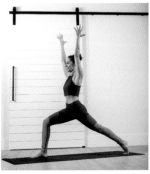

18 Step forward into crescent lunge on right side for 5 breaths
(page 124)

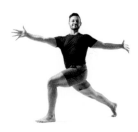

19 Open-arm crescent twist on right side for 5 breaths
(page 156)

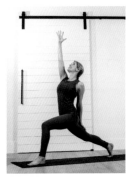

20 Reverse open-arm crescent twist on right side for 5 breaths
(page 156)

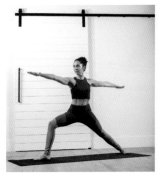

21 Warrior II on right side for 5 breaths
(page 117)

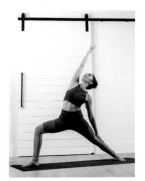

22 Reverse warrior on right side for 5 breaths
(page 118)

23 Vinyasa (page 98). Repeat steps 14-22 on the left side, then repeat steps again on both sides in a flow of one breath per movement.

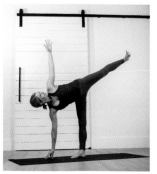

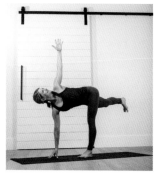

24 Balancing half moon on right side for 5 breaths
(page 148)

25 Revolved half moon on right side for 5 breaths
(page 149)

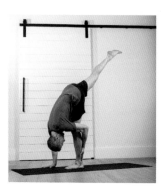

26 Standing splits on right side for 5 breaths
(page 151)

27 Vinyasa (page 98). Repeat on the left side, then repeat steps 14-26 two more times on each side in a flow at the pace of one breath per movement. On these last two rounds, balancing half moon is on an exhale and inhale, revolved half moon is on an exhale and inhale, and standing splits is on an exhale.

> continued

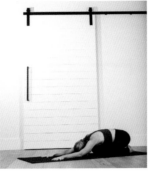

28 Child's pose for 10 breaths
(page 63)

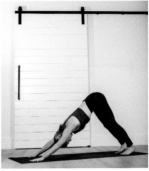

29 Downward-facing dog
for 5 breaths
(page 80)

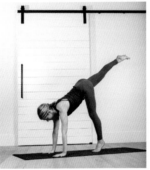

30 Handstand hops 5 times on
each side (prep shown)
(page 203)

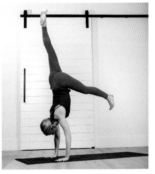

31 Handstand switch kicks
for 10 times
(page 203)

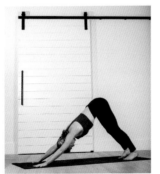

32 Downward-facing dog
for 5 breaths
(page 80)

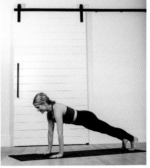

33 High plank, then slowly lower
to floor using 5 breaths
(page 85)

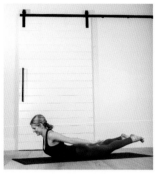

34 Locust for 5 breaths
(page 176)

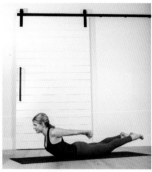

35 Locust with a bind for
5 breaths
(page 176)

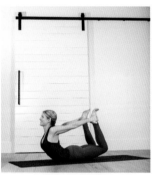

36 Floor bow for 2 rounds of
5 breaths each
(page 177)

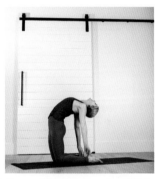

37 Camel for 2 rounds of 5 breaths
each (rest for 5 breaths in kneeling
position between each round)
(page 179)

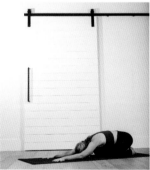

38 Child's pose for
10 breaths
(page 63)

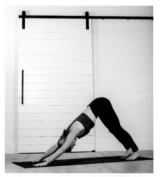

39 Downward-facing dog
for 5 breaths
(page 80)

> continued

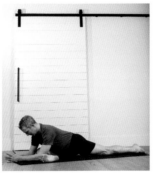

40 Half pigeon on right side
for 20 breaths
(page 224)

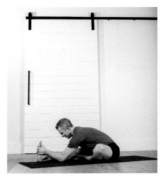

41 Single-leg forward fold with left
leg extended for 15 breaths
(page 236)

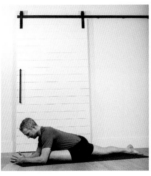

42 Half pigeon on left side
for 20 breaths
(page 224)

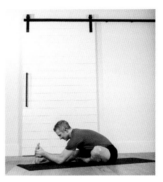

43 Single-leg forward fold with right
leg extended for 15 breaths
(page 236)

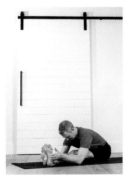

44 Seated forward
fold for 20 breaths
(page 235)

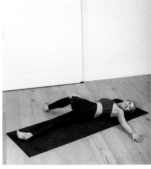

45 Supine twist for 10
breaths each side
(page 69)

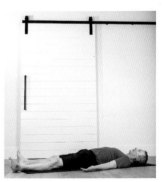

46 Final rest for 5 minutes
or more
(page 241)

You have the freedom to customize your practice using the blueprint for a power yoga class on page 316 and sequences outlined in the earlier chapters to create a plan that works for you. The sequences outlined in the previous chapters are like building blocks that you can plug in to the blueprint and use to create a holistic journey for your body and mind. This option gives you the permission and flexibility to adapt your practice depending on your needs, goals, and how you feel, and to use your intuition and inner wisdom to guide your practice. Follow the same progression, starting with 20 minutes of daily power yoga in the first week, 30 minutes in the second, 45 minutes in the third, and build to 60 minutes in the final week. The following are examples of how to build your own plan:

Build-Your-Own 20-Minute Sequence

Child's pose	5-minute lower-body sequence
2 Sun As	5-minute cooldown
2 Sun Bs	Rest

Build-Your-Own 30-Minute Sequence

Child's pose	10-minute upper-body sequence
3 Sun As	5-minute cooldown
3 Sun Bs	Rest
5-minute lower-body sequence	

Build-Your-Own 45-Minute Sequence

Child's pose	10-minute core sequence
5 Sun As	10 minutes of peak poses (backbends)
3 Sun Bs	10-minute cooldown
5-minute lower-body sequence	Rest

Build-Your-Own 60-Minute Sequence

Child's pose	15-minute lower-body sequence
5 Sun As	10 minutes of peak poses (backbends)
5 Sun Bs	10-minute cooldown
5-minute core sequence	Rest

Congratulations! You've completed your 28-day power yoga plan. You've done the work and taken the first steps on your transformative journey of power yoga. The practice is now in your bones, and your new power is flowing through your body, breath, and being. You get to move forward with the embodied wisdom of how to live and move with more power and purpose. You've experienced the uplifting results from your power yoga practice, and now you can choose what you keep

One becomes firmly established in practice only after attending to it for a long time, without interruption and with an attitude of devotion.

The Yoga Sutras of Patanjali:
Yoga Sutra 1.14

as you continue to practice and take the next steps of your yogic journey. This is just the beginning of your powerful way forward.

The techniques and practices of power yoga are not new. They are the essence of timeless transformational tools designed to empower your body, mind, and spirit. This book, these practices and sequences, and the ancient wisdom of yoga are always available for you to tap into. Power yoga is a daily opportunity to go beyond just a workout and access your greatest power and potential with one holistic practice.

Your power yoga practice gives you a way to unlock and unleash your power. When you are tapped into your personal power on the mat, you can carry your inner strength off the mat and use your power yoga practice to fuel your life.

On your journey forward, keep your eye on your why. There is no one way to practice yoga, and as you know by now, there is no right way to do any pose. Practice in a way that works for you, leave out what doesn't work, and find what feels good. You now have all the tools you need to continue to practice daily on your own, to add more challenge or advanced poses, or to find your tribe at a local yoga studio.

However you choose to expand your practice from here, may your yoga continue to empower you to be and feel your best. May your practice ignite your embodied wisdom and rich inner knowing. May you always know your power and be connected to your source and purpose. And may your power yoga practice be a tool for you to create and live a life of vibrancy, abundance, joy, and love. You deserve it all.

ABOUT THE AUTHOR

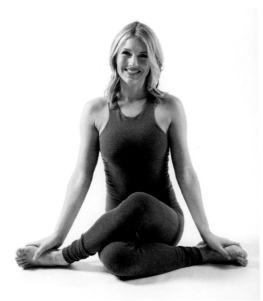

Leah Cullis, E-RYT 500, is a celebrated power yoga teacher and holistic health coach. She has worked with the Baptiste Institute and her teacher, world-renowned yogi and best-selling author Baron Baptiste, to design and deliver transformational power yoga programs. She has also studied under Jonny Kest and Lama Marut.

Cullis lives and teaches in Austin, TX, where she leads teacher trainings, workshops, and classes. She is the creator and leader of Pillars of Power Yoga, *Yoga Journal's* award-winning online course. She is a regular contributor to *Yoga Journal.*

Cullis is an all-star teacher with DoYouYoga.com, where she has created the Ultimate Guide to Power Yoga program and a free power yoga challenge that has been joined by 20,000 participants. She has been featured in *Mantra* Magazine, ElephantJournal.com, and Mind-BodyGreen.com. Cullis teaches at conferences and festivals across the country and has presented at prestigious institutions such as the Kripalu Center for Yoga and Health.

Cullis is a two-time ambassador for lululemon in Austin, Texas, and has represented her community at international conferences and retreats. From 2009 through 2016 she organized the Yoga Garden at the annual White House Easter Egg Roll, leading a team of nationally recognized teachers who shared yoga with more than 30,000 participants, as part of a presidential initiative encouraging healthy lifestyles for children and families. Her greatest honor is being a mom. Her website is http://leahcullis.com.

You read the book—now complete an exam to earn continuing education credit.

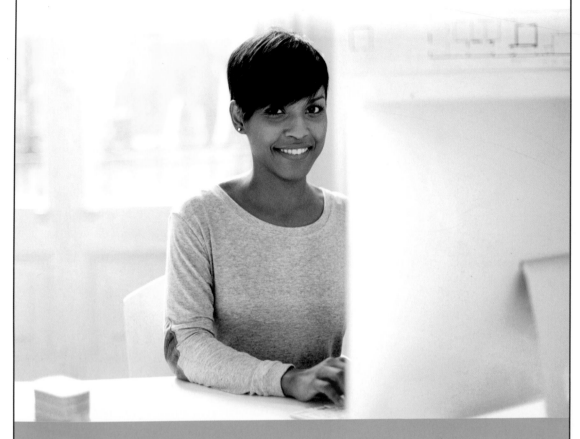

Congratulations on successfully preparing for this continuing education exam!

If you would like to earn CE credit, please visit

www.HumanKinetics.com/CE-Exam-Access

for complete instructions on how to access your exam.

Take advantage of a discounted rate by entering promo code **PY2019** when prompted.

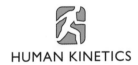

HUMAN KINETICS

6/18